SALICYLATE INTOLERANCE

SURVIVAL GUIDE

Theresa Cleaver *RGN RMN*

www.salicylate-intolerance.com

ACKNOWLEDGEMENT

Before embarking on this book, I had not realised that you would have to have such perseverance and dedication and many a time I questioned my ability to write one, especially when it went over 500 pages and threatened to go into another hemisphere, from my grey matter to dark matter and into a black hole.

Luckily help was at hand with my son Peter who laboriously and meticulously proofread it, so we have this final issue. My thanks to my daughter Aimee in her usual efficient expert way created the photos. To Anthony my son for his many inventive recipes with so few ingredients. To my husband who has said very little throughout the entire time I was writing this book possibly because he had some peace and quiet.

I'm eternally grateful to Moorfields Eye Hospital London who saved my eyesight, and also to my GP for his kindness and consideration over the years.

My thanks to my dear friend Lucy Crabtree a professional artist who created the illustrations exactly as I requested and beyond.

Most importantly I want to thank God for his steadfast love because without him this book would never have happened, and I pray you find healing.

Charles Dickens

"Reflect upon your present blessings, of which every man has plenty.

not on your past misfortunes, of which all men have some."

Peter Cleaver www.petercleavermusic.co.uk

Aimee Cleaver www.aimeecleaver.co.uk

Lucy Crabtree www.lucycrabtreeart.com

IMPORTANT INFORMATION TO READ

You are responsible for your own wellness and safety at all times.

The contents of this book are designed to provide helpful information on Salicylate intolerance and is current and accurate at the time of publication. This book is not meant to be used, to diagnose or treat any medical condition. Always seek the advice of your physician or other qualified health provider with any questions you may have regarding a medical condition. Never ignore professional medical advice or delay in seeking it.

Dietary intervention, whether for the purposes of diagnosis under a Doctor's supervision or management of food intolerance, needs a suitably trained dietitian to ensure nutritional needs are met. This is particularly true if you suffer from diabetes.

This book lists foods that I can take without an adverse reaction – it is what works for me – it is not a definitive list of what you can eat. For instance, some people can cope with moderate amounts of Salicylates with no ill effect.

You should also be aware of the following: -

In different English-speaking nations, the same food can hold different names and the same name can refer to different foods, for example what Australians call shallots, English people call salad onions. Farming and processing methods may affect the salicylate content of a food. Research into the salicylate content of different foods is on-going. This means that the recorded level of salicylates in foods such as fruit, vegetables and herbs have been changed periodically in the past and may change in the future depending on the results of new research. For example, parsley used to be rated as low in Salicylate but recent research now rates parsley as moderate. Similarly, golden delicious apples on some lists has gone from low to moderate so you need to be constantly vigilant and checking labels. The ingredients list on food packaging changes over time as manufacturers are constantly tweaking their recipes.

References are provided for informational purposes only and do not constitute endorsement of any websites or other sources.

CONTENTS

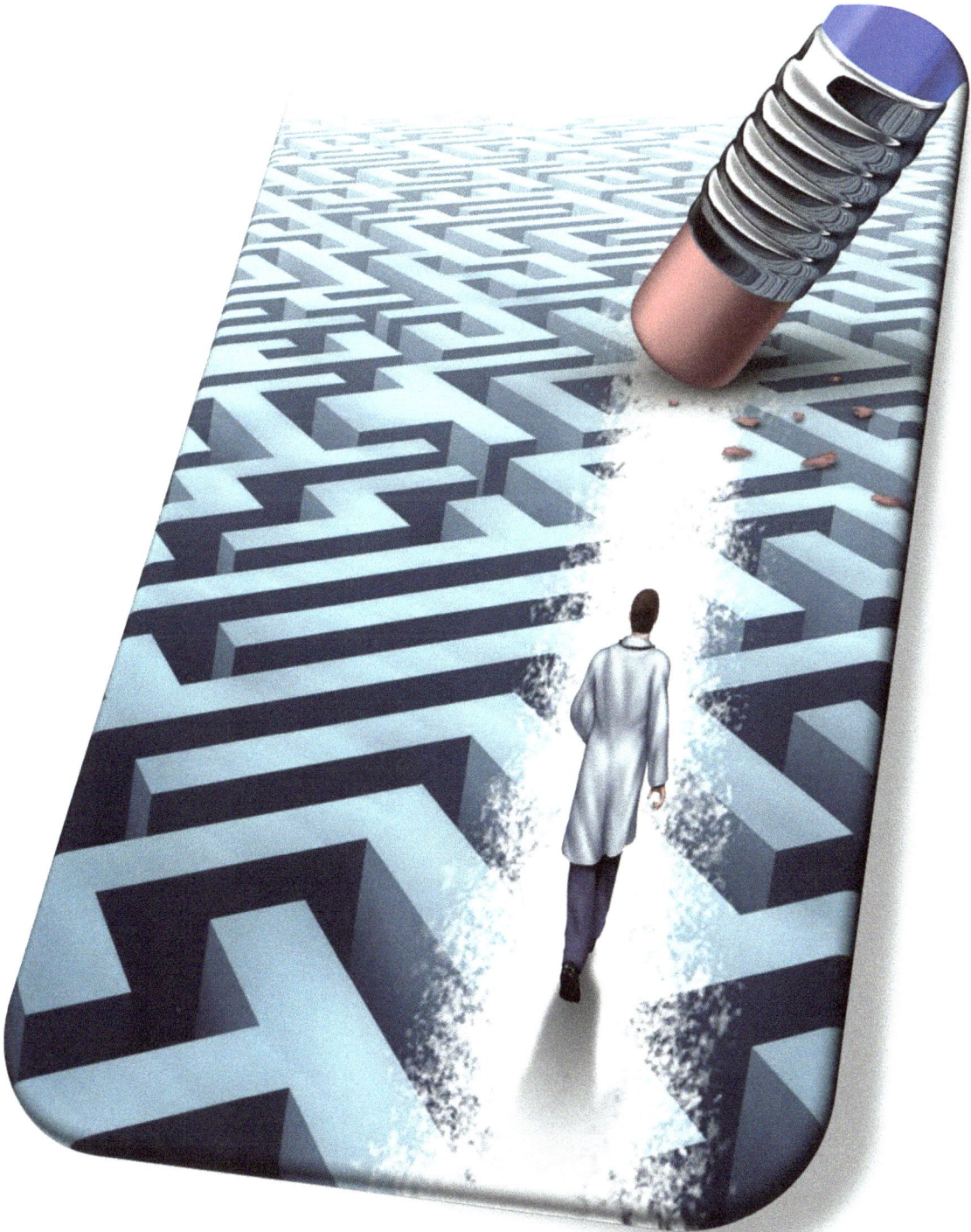

SALICYLATE INTOLERANCE

A LONG-CONVOLUTED ROAD

TO DIAGNOSIS

When I was at my weakest, I had to be at my strongest to find a cure.

Manufacturers change the ingredients used frequently and use vague terms

such as vegetable' oil and natural flavourings.

THE LONG-CONVOLUTED ROAD TO DIAGNOSIS

When I started having allergic type symptoms without any sign of a diagnoses, it was fortunate that I was dual qualified Nurse in psychiatry and general, so could use my training to find a solution. In May 2005 after switching to a new eye cream I developed swollen red eyes, which I promptly stopped but the symptoms remained. Still, after studying the ingredients they contained salicylic acid, which is the same as aspirin, which I am allergic to. Months afterwards, it was one of the key clues towards bringing a diagnosis.

At first, as I suffered from Hay fever, I assumed this was the cause, but by September my face was fully swollen, which no amount of hay fever medications could rectify. Through early Autumn I was very toxic, my hands were shaking, I was vomiting profusely daily and found myself hyperactive throughout all hours (leading me to bake cookies for the children in the night – something they certainly appreciated). Plus, within just six weeks, I dropped down from size 14 to a size 6 in clothes!

My health was rapidly deteriorating, I was exhausted, haggard and frustrated at the total lack of interest in finding a causal factor for the swelling which every doctor I saw was putting it down to unknown allergy causes (idiopathic allergy). I even went to a private allergist consultant who, after a hefty payment gave the broad diagnosis of "I've seen worse". The straw that broke the camel's back was when a Doctor, inferred I should just live with it and take antihistamines. I told him I was seriously ill and that I would get the solution myself.

Research - How it developed

I already knew I had two known allergies hay fever and aspirin. Many years before while on duty I had a sore throat, and I was advised to gargle with aspirin which promptly developed into full blown allergic reaction with a rash and swollen face. Fortunately, it happened while I was giving the report, as I was swiftly given antihistamines. Afterwards, the medical staff thanked me for a first-hand experience of the stages of an allergic reaction! So, knowing I was already allergic to Aspirin (salicylic acid), and as facial swelling is a key sign, I figured that it seemed a good place to start my research. I found that salicylates were also in food -fruit and vegetables. I realised I had recently altered my diet and I was eating for the first-time curries and apple pie with nutmeg both of which have high salicylates.

By December 2005, I had concluded that I had salicylate intolerance. I made an appointment with a kind doctor specialising in allergies in Harley Street who after some tests confirmed salicylate intolerance. It appeared in rare cases salicylate intolerance can occur from an aspirin allergy as they are both salicylates.

Still, I was ecstatic to finally have a diagnosis because now I could go forward and become well. The allergist also suggested a thyroid function test which was dangerously high (T4 60 and I was on the brink of collapse) and this led to the diagnosis of the Graves' disease. Put simply my own immune system was overloaded and fighting against itself, perhaps stimulated by the high levels of salicylates causing toxicity.

ALLERGIC REACTIONS

When I was a student nurse in psychiatry, I developed a mysterious rash with severe skin peeling which took several weeks to clear but never recurred. During this episode while at a nursing class, I noticed a glove on the desk, just for me to realise it was my discarded skin! My colleagues jokingly decided I was either a snake or had leprosy and gave me a bell to ring whenever I was about.

In recent years I have received a few severe allergic reactions not all are named here. One was possibly due to chemicals in a London experience event where they suggested we place our hands in a solution and see it glow and without thinking I dipped in one finger (I know we never learn). My daughter duly marched me off to wash my hands (how the tables turn). However, once I got home, I noticed my face was swollen (angioedema), and I was finding it difficult to swallow which resulted in a trip to A&E and high dose of steroids for some weeks.

Shopping Mall are a problem as I have been caught out a few times so that now I avoid them. Once I went into a shop just after they let people back in after a fire alert, I noticed some strong sweet smells perhaps to cover something up and again ended up on high steroids. Most people will have milder reactions to salicylates but the combination of being allergic to Aspirin and having an autoimmune disease may have precipitated my reactions.

Potential triggers for salicylate intolerance

High levels of stress especially those genetically predisposed to certain illness are known to activate many diseases.

In 2004 for the first ever I started eating curries and apple pies with nutmeg both of which are high in salicylates. Another potential trigger could have been that in January 2005 a family member died. The same week I underwent a major surgical procedure. By May I began displaying symptoms.

Reducing Toxins: The consultant who diagnosed Salicylate intolerance gave me a short list of foods to avoid, mainly high salicylates and tartrazine and benzoic acid and I made very little progress. Persevering, I lived on a strict low salicylate diet for several weeks and this started the road to recovery and while I was still far from the model of health, I felt better than I had for infinity! Through my research I discovered that salicylates were everywhere, from the foods we eat, to the soaps we use. As a countermeasure, I scrutinised all food ingredient labels and avoided perfumes and cleaning chemicals and lots more. Details of which are in other chapters.

Broadly speaking, I have good days and bad and I am blessed with a very understanding family that keep me on track when I nearly succumb to a yummy dessert that tempts me! Hopefully, your reactions will be milder, so don't be discouraged, the whole aim of this book is to help you understand your condition better and to make it easier to go through the mirage of information out there. Unfortunately, some medical professional may know little or nothing about salicylate intolerance because it remains a rare condition with very little research done to date.

SOURCE: Autoimmune disease https://www.nap.edu/read/1591/chapter/6#60. Xenobiotics exposures can induce autoimmune disorders, which sometimes require a genetic predisposition. Very little research has been done so that and we do not know the extent to which apparently spontaneous autoimmune disorders are influenced by environmental factors.

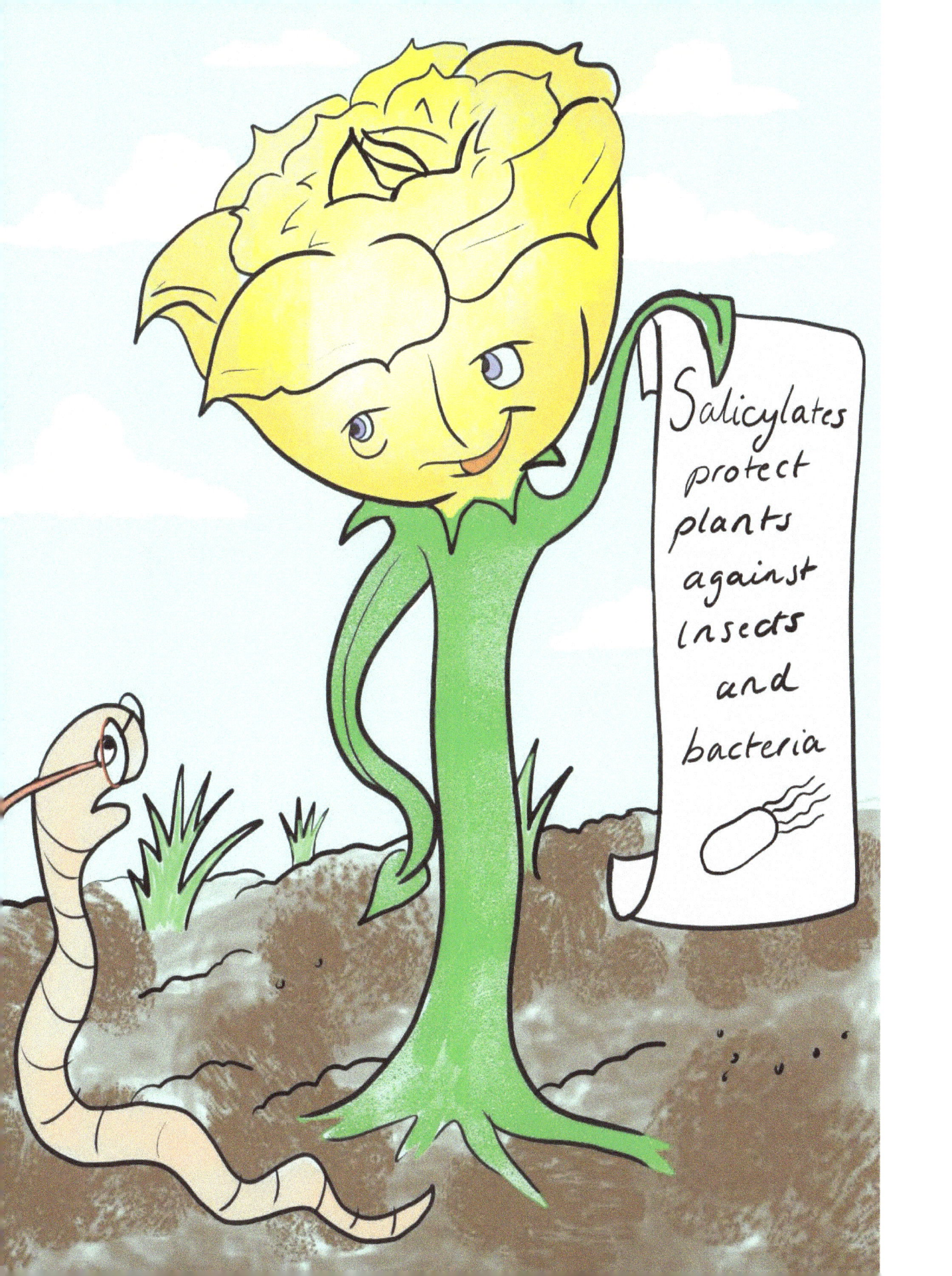

Salicylates protect plants against insects and bacteria

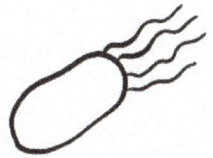

NATURAL & ARTIFICIAL CHEMICALS

Salicylates- SALICYLIC ACID

Aspirin

The salts and esters of salicylic acid are known as salicylates

Salicylate intolerance mimics Aspirin symptoms

because the mechanism of action of these substances is quite similar.

NATURAL AND ARTIFICIAL SALICYLATES

If you react to salicylates, you will react to naturally occurring food chemicals, and synthetic additives such as food colourings, flavour enhancers and preservatives.

Chemicals are prevalent in our world even, our bodies are chemical factories where there are hundreds of internal secretions, enzymes, proteins. Naturally chemicals can be mined out of the earth such as carbon, oil, and coal, or refined from living organisms such as animals or plants.

Man-made chemicals are manufactured and can be identical to natural chemicals, for example, natural vitamin C (ascorbic acid) from fruits, can be synthesized from glucose and the product is the same as the naturally occurring substance.

Ever since the 16th century, both natural and artificial chemicals have been known to be life-threatening depending on its concentration, so the dosage is really the key factor here. For example, natural chemicals that can be toxic: cyanide occurs naturally in certain foods and from these natural sources it is not necessarily toxic. It is the concentration that makes cyanide lethal.

What are salicylates?

Salicylates are a group of chemicals derived from salicylic acid. Salicylate is a natural chemical found in plants which use it as a preservative to protect themselves against disease, bacteria fungi and insects.

What is Salicylic acid (2-Hydroxybenzoic acid)

Salicylic acid is derived from the metabolism of salicin and is a naturally occurring phenol. It functions as a plant hormone to determine growth, development and a defence system against diseases, worms, bacteria, and environmental stress.

Salicylates, including salicin and salicylic acid, are found in the bark and leaves of the willow and poplar trees. The leaves of the willow tree have been used for medicinal purposes to reduce fever and pain since antiquity. However, by the 1900 it was synthesised and given the brand name Aspirin.

Natural Salicylates

They are found naturally in certain foods for example fruit and vegetables have salicylates in them. Other natural sources are Wintergreen which is produced from the leaves of that plant. They are made into wintergreen oil, methyl salicylate, which is closely related to aspirin and has analgesic and anti-inflammatory properties. These are high in salicylates and are best avoided.

Synthetic Salicylates

Salicylic acid can be synthesised to be used as an ingredient in medicines (most notably aspirin), shampoos, personal care products, cleaning products, and as a preservative.

Salicylate in plant-based food is lower when compared taking a moderate dose of aspirin.

SALICYLATES

Salicylate food chemicals and amines accumulate in the system sometimes over several days causing symptoms. Also, some individuals may also react to smells and fumes in the environment.

Food & Environment Salicylates are found in most foods, artificial preservatives, colourings, flavourings and in the environment, which makes them difficult to avoid. Food chemicals can cause a cumulative toxic effect and contribute to illness.

Treatment: is avoidance of triggers and low salicylate diet to reduce build up leading to symptoms. (See chapter)

Salicylates Intolerance and other chemicals that may cause reactions. Phenols (benzene ring structure) Both phenol and *salicylates are chemically similar* because they are based on a benzene ring structure. Nearly all foods have phenols, but in different quantities.

Amines Those with salicylate Intolerance often are intolerant of amines. The symptoms of amine intolerance are similar to salicylate intolerance, which can make it difficult to differentiate.

Benzoates (benzene ring structure) The salts and esters of benzoic acid are known as Benzoates. Some propose a cross over reaction to those who have a salicylate Intolerance with similar symptoms.

Tartrazine (colouring) With salicylate Intolerance you also react to tartrazine possibly due to the fact they are detoxified by the same elimination pathway in the body.

Sulphates Those low in sulphate are likely to react to salicylates, food colours and other additives.

Nitrites these are found in many food colourings and flavourings are chemically similar to salicylates.

Mono Sodium Glutamate (sodium glutamate) Is a flavour enhancer commonly added to Chinese food, canned vegetables, soups and processed meats and may also cause similar reaction as salicylates.

MAN MADE SALICYLATES

Salicylates intolerance mimics Aspirin symptoms, rarely those allergic to aspirin developed salicylate intolerance

Salicylate Intolerance and Aspirin

Seldom, people who are allergic to aspirin will react if they have foods that have high levels of natural salicylates.

However, if you have salicylate intolerance you must avoid aspirin as it is salicylates acid and will accumulate in the blood causing symptoms. Although rare, I suffer from both aspirin allergy and salicylates intolerance.

Reaction to ingredients like Salicylates

Upwards to 25% of people who are hypersensitive to aspirin also react to the azo dye tartrazine, Benzoates, and sulphites.

The symptoms are often indistinguishable from those resulting from salicylate intolerance because the mechanism of action of these substances is quite similar. For this reason, these ingredients should therefore be avoided.

ASPIRIN

Aspirin - medically known as acetylsalicylic acid was first manufactured in 1899 from the willow plant, but the leaves were used since ancient times as a pain killer. Aspirin is a well-known derivative of salicylic acid and the word salicylate refers to the active ingredient in the drugs. Aspirin works by being taken up into the blood flow from the upper small intestine and once there converts into salicylic acid. It helps reduce pain, swelling, fever and can also help reduce the risk of heart attacks and certain strokes by taking a small, prescribed dose daily to thin the blood and prevent clots.

Aspirin Allergy

Some people are truly allergic to aspirin, while others are intolerant. Allergic reactions show up with an antibody in the blood test (Immunoglobulin E) whilst those intolerants will not have this antibody in the blood. Aspirin allergy symptoms range from mild to severe, occurring within minutes to hours of taking the medication. Diagnosis is determined by the reaction and symptoms after ingestion of Aspirin.

Symptoms are hives, itchy skin, runny nose, reddish eyes, welling up of either the lips, tongue, or face, coughing, wheezing or shortness of breath, or even anaphylaxis — a rare, severe allergic reaction and demands prompt medical treatment. If you react to Aspirin you need to avoid medication that are closely related to aspirin, such as Ibuprofen, Nurofen etc...

Those diagnosed sensitive to Aspirin are not necessary sensitivity to salicylate in foods Please observe it is worth understanding Aspirin to understand Salicylate Intolerance.

ASPIRIN POISONING (Salicylism)

This is often caused from taking an excessive amount of Aspirin or oil of wintergreen (small amounts can be toxic) either accidentally such as with children or adults who take Aspirin alongside other medication that also has Aspirin in them. Symptoms range from mild reactions, like ringing in the ears, nausea, and vomiting to severe confusion, hyperventilation, seizures, or can even lead to a coma.

Treatment: Initially, activated charcoal is given which adsorbs the aspirin in the gastrointestinal tract. Stomach pumping is only done if lethal amounts have been taken less than one-hour previously. Intravenous (fluids into the arm) fluids of sodium bicarbonate are given in a significant aspirin overdose.

Three phases of toxicity (*More Salicylates and detoxification*)

Phase I: Respiratory alkalosis (duration 12 hours) This is characterized by hyperventilation. The body compensates by the urine becoming alkaline (urine usually slightly acidic). Potassium and sodium bicarbonate are excreted in the urine at this stage.

Phase II: Metabolic acidosis (duration 12/ 24 hours) Respiratory alkalosis leads to increase of acid in the urine. Due to this, the kidneys are unable to effectively neutralize the effects of the acid, which lead to a reduction in bicarbonate formation.

Phase III: Severe metabolic acidosis (duration 24 hours) The pH of blood ranges from 7.35-7.45, (pH of other body fluids is different). Progressive metabolic acidosis leads to low blood pH (less than 7.35 - due to the inability of the body to form bicarbonate in the kidney. This leads to dehydration, and deficiency of potassium in the bloodstream and has serious consequences, leading to coma or even death.

Chronic toxicity: this can develop from doses of aspirin at 100 mg/kg/day in people. Especially true in the elderly (De Groen, 1989) who may consume an increasing amount over several days causing confusion

SOURCE Salicylate Poisoning (Diagnosis and Management) http://www.you tube.com/ watch=2HK_TWArXiQ

VARIOUS TYPES OF SALICYLATES

Acetylsalicylic acid- (Aspirin)

Benzoates

Benzoyl salicylate

Beta-hydroxyl acid -BHA

Butylated hydroxytoluene-BHT

Choline salicylate -(NSAID)

Ethyl Salicylate--perfumery and artificial flavours

Isooctyl salicylate - flavouring agent

Isoamyl salicylate-flavour and fragrance agents

Magnesium salicylate

Methyl Salicylate - (oil of wintergreen)

Mono sodium salicylate

Octyl Salicylate - sunscreens and cosmetics

Phenyl Salicylate -polymers, lacquers, adhesives, waxes, and polishes

Phenyl ethyl salicylate

Salicylic Acid

Salicylaldehyde

Salicylamide -pain killer

Salsalate -pain killer

Sodium Salicylate

Some Salicylate-Containing Ingredients

TYPES OF SALICYLATES cont

Aloe Vera

Artificial flavourings Artificial food

colourings Azo dyes

Coal tar dyes

Disalcid

Eucalyptus Oil Menthol

Mint

Nitrates

Nitrites

Peppermint

Red Dye

Spearmint

Yellow Dye

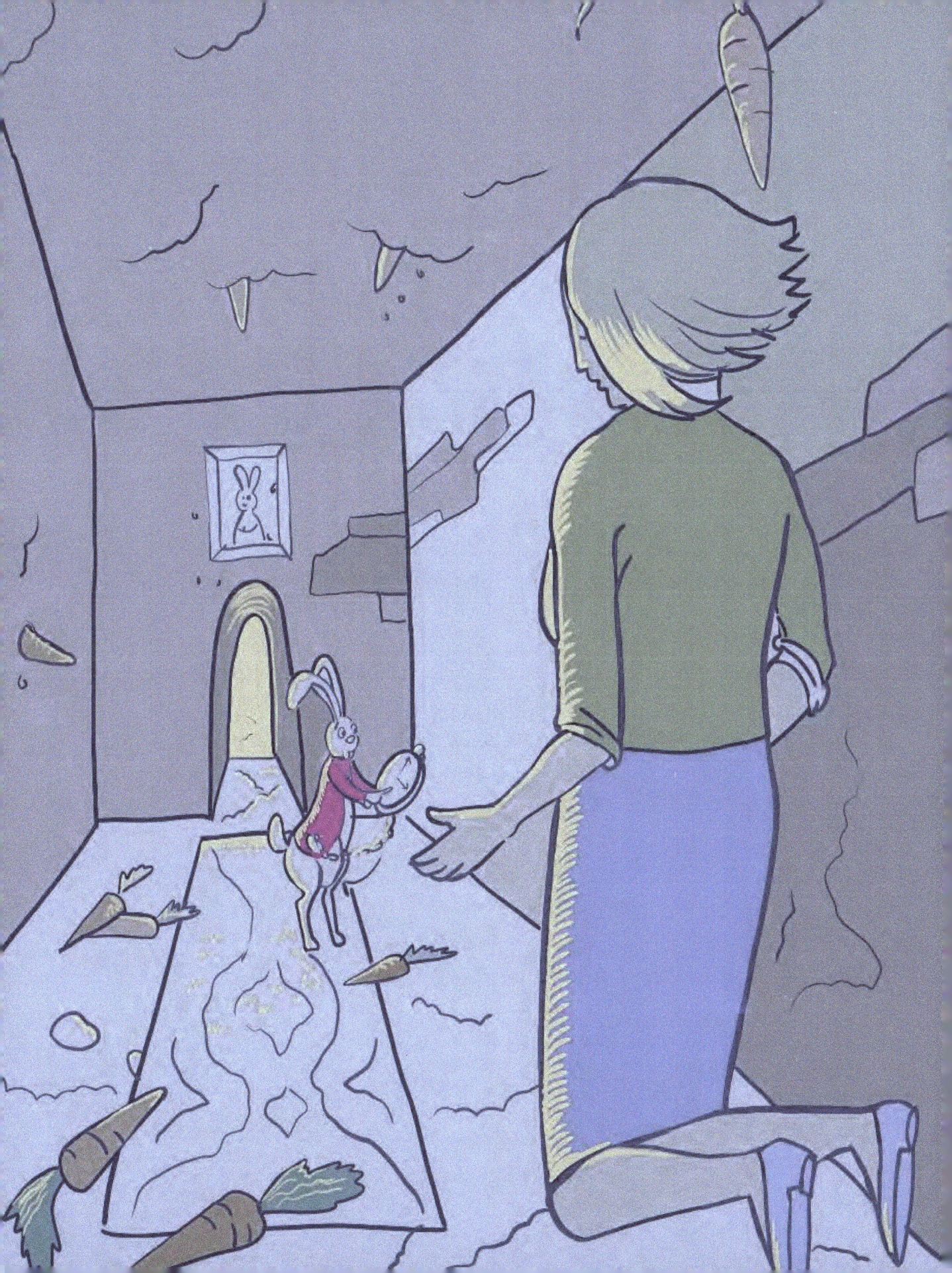

FOOD INTOLERANCE & ALLERGY

SEARCHING FOR ANSWERS

Food intolerance can be mistaken for food allergy

FOOD INTOLERANCE & FOOD ALLERGY

Food intolerance is chronic with variable symptoms and can be mistaken for the symptoms of a food allergy.

A food intolerance causes problems digesting certain foods, whilst food allergies respond to a food protein and affects the immune system.

FOOD ALLERGY *Food allergic reactions can run in families.*

In susceptible people with food allergy happens when your immune system perceives harmless proteins in certain foods as a threat and produces antibodies called Immunoglobulin E (IgE), resulting in an allergic response. This results in the releases of histamine in the body, causing an inflammatory response and symptoms. Responses can be serious enough to be life threatening (anaphylaxis). Some of the common food allergies are nuts, dairy products, soybean, wheat, seafood, eggs, sesame.

Symptoms: food allergies can be immediate or up to two hours after ingestion of food and can cause symptoms such as swelling of face, mouth and throat, trouble breathing, abdominal pain, nausea or vomiting, rashes (hives).

Anaphylactic: this is a medical emergency which causes difficulty in breathing (throat swelling), feeling faint (blood pressure dropping) and is treated with adrenaline injection such as an EpiPen auto injector. (*see chart*)

Test for food allergies: Skin prick tests and blood tests.

Phenol Intolerance/Allergy

Phenolic compounds are everywhere and very difficult to avoid. An allergic reaction happens when your body mistakes phenol compounds as a threat and releases histamines and other chemicals into the body causing symptoms.

People who consume large amounts of foods high in phenol or foods containing salicylates and additives may experience symptoms (similar to salicylate intolerance).

The response can be a runny nose, dark circles under the eyes, reddened eyes, wheezing, digestive issues or even pain, rash, and other skin conditions.

Low phenol diet: reactions from phenols can cause mild depression and lassitude, and symptoms may worsen with stress. Still, avoiding the higher levels of phenols and eliminating artificial colours and flavours should help to alleviate some symptoms and antihistamine help.

Salicylates are not allergens(proteins) and they do not trigger a response of the immune system, and therefore, cannot induce an anaphylactic reaction. Aspirin is the only known salicylate to cause an allergic reaction and anaphylaxis. Some allergies such as hay fever do not cause any lasting problems whereas nuts can be - life threatening leading to Anaphylaxis.

FOOD INTOLERANCE

Food Intolerance also known as non-IgE mediated or non-allergic food hypersensitivity. Food intolerance affects the digestive system and can result from the absence of specific chemicals or enzymes needed to digest food. It can also occur to natural chemicals in foods, as in salicylate intolerance.

List of food intolerance include:

Salicylate intolerance: occurs when normal amounts of ingested natural salicylate found in fruit and vegetables, processed foods with flavour additives cause a response.

Lactose intolerance: this occurs when the body is unable to digest lactose, a type of sugar in milk and dairy product and is due to absence or deficiency of an enzyme.

Amines intolerance: (cause pharmacological reactions), found in foods and beverages.

Sulphites intolerance: sensitivity to food additives.

Histamine intolerance: natural histamine in some foods.

MSG intolerance (mono sodium glutamate): flavour enhancers.

Caffeine intolerance: coffee, tea, chocolates.

Symptoms: food Intolerance reactions may be immediate or up to 48 hours such as abdominal pain, nausea, vomiting, hives, headaches. You can keep a diary of offending foods and eliminate them from your diet.

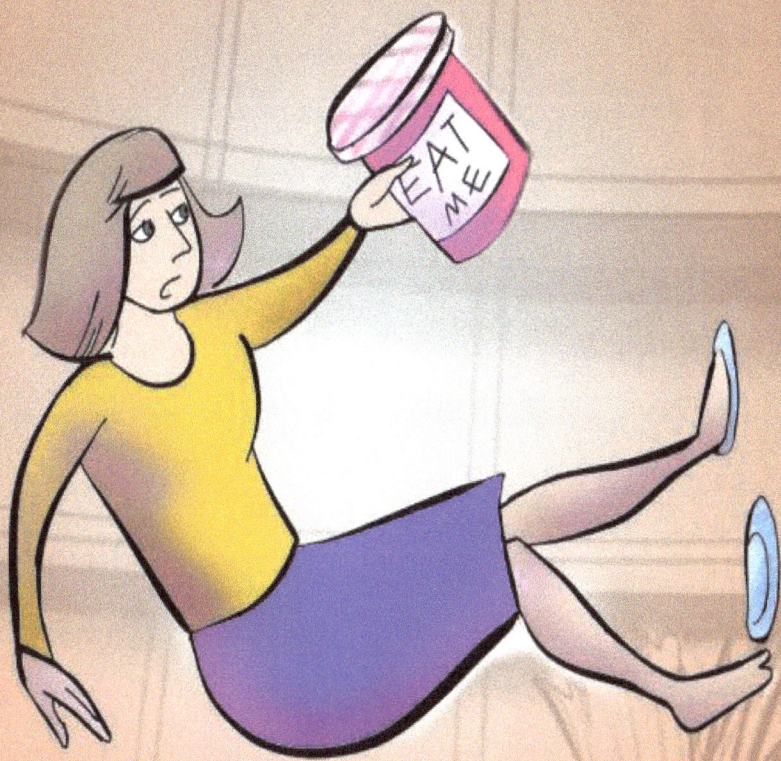

SALICYLATE INTOLERANCE

"Salicylate intolerance is defined as a non-specific antigen-induced pseudo-allergic hypersensitivity reaction which can occur upon contact of an organism with salicylic acid, its derivatives or other related organic or inorganic acids of similar chemical structure".

Salicylate absorbed through, ingestion, inhaled, the skin or all three.

SALICYLATE INTOLERANCE

If you react to salicylates, you are more probable to also be sensitive to other naturally occurring food chemicals (such as amines and glutamate), and to synthetic additives such as food colourings, flavour enhancers and preservatives. Although reactions to salicylate has been known for more than 100 years, it is not adequately recognised in the relevant areas of medicine. In large amounts, salicylates are poisonous to everyone, but for those who suffer from salicylate intolerance, even a small amount can overwhelm the body especially at the beginning.

What is Salicylate Intolerance

The symptoms of salicylate intolerance are often misinterpreted as allergies. Salicylate intolerance is when the body reacts to salicylates, but it does not involve the immune system. A salicylate sensitive person may have difficulty tolerating certain fruits, vegetables, or any products that contain aspirin. For some they will react to, ingested, inhaled or through the skin or all three. Others may just experience a reaction to high doses of salicylates. Some may notice over time that they can tolerate more salicylate without problems, while others may always be susceptible even to small amount and I am one of those people. By choosing a low salicylate diet at first you can reduce the symptoms. A low salicylate diet means that you carefully eat foods that contain no salicylate or low in salicylate, and you avoid high salicylate food.

Salicylate Intolerance differs from salicylism (excessive intake of salicylates) which is mostly due to excessive intake of salicylic acid, mainly aspirin or its derivatives. There are no laboratory or skin testing methods for testing salicylate intolerance and the only way to find out is by having an elimination diet of all high salicylates and see if there is an improvement.

Symptoms of Salicylate Intolerance Some people have symptoms after ingestion of a minuscule quantity of these chemicals, while others can tolerate larger amounts before a reaction is triggered.

LIST OF SYMPTOMS SALICYLATE INTOLERANCE

Here are the symptoms I sometimes experience- See link at bottom of this page for other symptoms.

Digestive: stomach pain, nausea, vomiting, flatulence, constipation. I respond to the ingestion of salicylate within 20 minutes to 8 hours later with profuse vomiting.

Respiratory: sinusitis/nasal polyps, cough, rarely difficulty in breathing. Coughing is usually due to environmental salicylates for example air fresheners and incense.

Skin: hives or rashes, changes in skin colour/skin discoloration. In mild case this clears on its own quite quickly

Eyes: sore, itchy, puffy, or burning eyes, dark circles under the eyes.

Ears: tinnitus ringing of the ears.

Joints: general aches and pains temporarily in joints.

Angioedema: I have had several bad attacks treated with steroids. I also have frequent mild facial swelling which clear within a few days without treatment.

Chronic fatigue: I can start the day feeling fine and then suddenly dip and find it hard to manage the smallest chore. Even so, usually it clears within a few hour's but sometimes may last for a couple of days and because of this my concentration can be low.

Allergens are proteins that trigger an immunological response with the production of antibodies. Salicylates are not allergens and thus do not trigger a response of the immune system and cannot induce an anaphylactic response.

SOURCE: *Symptoms of Salicylate Sensitivity / Salicylate Intolerance? http://salicylatesensitivity.com/info3/. Salicylate Intolerance Pathophysiology, Clinical Spectrum, Diagnosis and Treatment. Https://www.ncbi.nlm.nih.gov/pmc/articles/PMC2696737/*

TRIGGERS OF SALICYLATE INTOLERANCE

Leukotrienes: Some research suggests Salicylate Intolerance may be due to an overproduction of leukotrienes. When the body encounters an allergen (usually a harmless substance), inflammatory chemicals are released into the body causing symptoms. Leukotrienes are involved in asthma, hay fever (allergic rhinitis) and allergic reactions and act to sustain inflammatory reactions.

This overproduction is caused by the inhibition of an enzyme (known as cyclooxygenase) that regulates the production of leukotrienes. This increase of leukotrienes in the body leads to symptoms related to salicylate intolerance.

Enzyme: insufficient amounts of a certain enzyme used to metabolise salicylates causing salicylates to accumulate in the body leading to a reaction.

Food additives: salicylates are sometimes used for substance added to food to enhance its flavour or appearance or to preserve it such as benzoic acid and tartrazine.

Stress response: When dealing with a stressful experience, the glands just above your kidneys known as the adrenal gland combat the negative effects that stress have on your body by producing the hormone cortisol. If the constant production of cortisol is left unchecked, this leads to what is known as adrenal exhaustion, which can lead to the symptoms of Salicylate intolerance.

Menopause: Women in their early 50s have a reduction of the hormone oestrogen and rarely this is thought to precipitate allergies and intolerances.

Bacterial invasion: when the immune defence system is lowered this may cause toxins to build up due to sluggish response.

SOURCE: Sensitivity to food additives, amines and salicylates: a review of the evidence, https://ctajournal.biomedcentral.com/articles/10.1186/s13601-015-0078-3. The difference diagnosis of food intolerance -Yurdagül Zopf, Dr. med https://www.ncbi.nlm.nih.gov/pmc/articles/PMC2695393/. Salicylate Intolerance -Diagnosis and Treatment -Hanns-

CHEMICAL THRESHOLD REACTION FOR SALICYLATE INTOLERANCE

I can only be able to tolerate small amounts before either vomiting or feeling toxic

How Salicylates are absorbed through the body

Digestive system: after ingestion of salicylates in foods the stomach lining becomes inflamed allowing molecules of protein, toxins, and other matter to pass through into the blood stream and then the immune system reacts by producing symptoms. These salicylates are distributed in joints, spinal fluid, and saliva but are at its lowest in the brain and skeletal tissue.

Skin Contact: salicylates are readily taken up through the skin from ointments, creams, oil of wintergreen, deep heat ointments, especially in treatments for warts.

Respiratory: inhaling salicylates from the environment such as incense and so forth.

Effects of Salicylates Intolerance on the body

These reactions depend on whether the salicylate is a portion of food, medicine, or others as well as the quantity ingested. Toxins accumulate, causing higher than normal levels of these chemicals in the blood and even a small amount may just tilt the balance and cause a reaction. Reaction times vary with everyone occurring from 30 minutes to 48 hours and even several days later after exposure.

Levels of salicylate in food may change because:

Soil: if it is grown in organic soil higher levels of salicylates often occur

Different standards: animal feed, fertilisers, processing can all affect salicylate levels

Ripeness: levels decreases the riper the fruit & vegetables are.

High levels of salicylates are found in the skin of fruit and vegetables so remove before eating it. Potatoes and pears, for instance, have salicylate but only in their skin.

Salicylate medication Those with salicylate intolerance often react adversely to medicines. Tell your doctor or pharmacist before taking any medication and check labels yourself before use. Some pills have flavourings and hidden salicylate such as phenol preservatives (BHA, BHT), benzoic acid, tartrazine colours.

Dentist: If they ask to employ an anaesthetic it is advisable for them to use plain Lignocaine as there are preservatives in alternatives.

Salicylate toxicity-Salicylism, see chapter. Some research indicates that those with salicylate Intolerance may be more susceptible to salicylate toxicity, as this occurs when the body's acid buffering systems are overloaded and overwhelmed leading to symptoms mimicking aspirin toxicity (ringing in the ears, nausea and so on). It is treated by limiting the absorption of salicylates.

Cholesterol synthesis

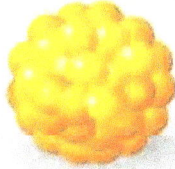

Help the absorption
of vitamins

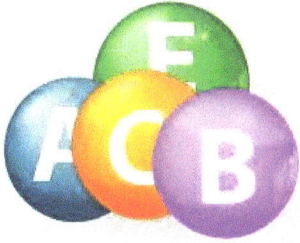

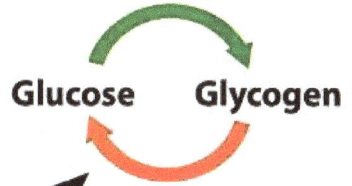

E
A C B

Glucose   Glycogen

Deactivation of
poisons and toxins

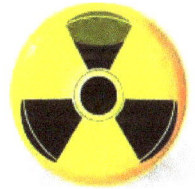

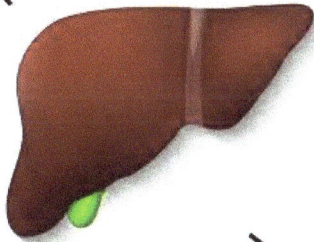

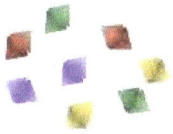

Hormones & enzymes
production and
detoxification

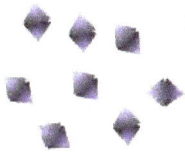

Produces
bile

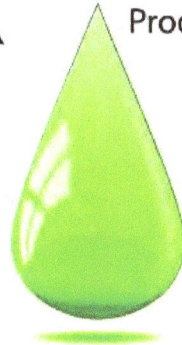

Amino acid synthesis

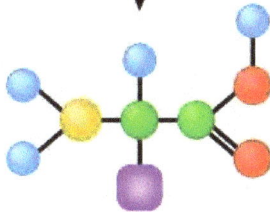

DETOXIFICATION

SALICYLATES

Phenols and Salicylates are metabolised by an enzyme phenol sulfotransferase (PST)

For detoxification to take place, our bodies must make sulphate

THE MECHANISM OF THE BODY'S DETOXIFICATION

Salicylate Intolerance detoxification system

Normally our body is well-equipped to eliminate toxins, but with salicylate Intolerance, toxins build up in the system causing symptoms.

It is helpful to realize the mechanism behind detoxification to help your recovery.

We exist in a universe full of toxins, and if our body is unable to process these toxins and excrete them; it results in a toxin build-up causing vomiting and other symptoms.

Detoxification, or detox, generally refers to the process of getting rid of toxins from the body. Our bodies accumulate toxins every day from the food we eat to the air we breathe, and the levels of toxins vary from person-to-person.

The body's natural detoxification process is dependent on the power of water to act as a solvent to break up toxic substances. We are constructed of approximately 75% water (of this % your brain is 80%!) so none of your body systems can work at the optimum level if you are dehydrated.

How effective the detoxification process is depending on what enzymes we have (inherited /genetics), and our intake of nutrients in our diet such as vitamins and amount of fluids we drink.

Types of Toxins

Xenobiotics: These are common environmental toxins and prescription drugs

Endobiotic: These are toxins produced within the body such as excess hormones, free radicals, and bile acids.

How the body works to eliminate toxins

The liver is a major organ for, digestion, energy storage, hormone production and is essential for detoxifying the body. When we are exposed to many toxins this slows down the liver process, causing an increase of toxins.

Regions of high levels of fatty tissues are the area where you will see the most toxins, for example, the brain, breast, and adrenal glands.

Toxins are mainly processed and rejected through the liver, but also through the kidneys, bowels, lungs, lymphatic system, and skin. If nutrition is compromised through poor dietary and lifestyle habits, the detoxification process will be impaired. The liver acts as a critical part in detox and the pace at which the liver can do away with toxins can determine susceptibility to toxic overload, which in turn can contribute to symptoms of poor health.

FACTORS THAT AID DETOXIFICATION PROCESS

Bile Rd. is made by the liver and it is stored in the gallbladder. It helps flush out the toxins from your body and is critical for dietary fats absorption and digestion. It plays a major role in moving toxins out of the liver and into the intestines, where they can be excreted out of the body.

Enzymes

Enzymes are proteins that help speed up chemical reactions in the human body without being consumed or permanently altered themselves. They are essential for respiration, digesting food, muscle tissue and nerve function. In detoxification they speed up a chemical response in the liver, making drugs and toxins into less toxic forms that are easier for the body to excrete. Most of the food we eat is complex carbohydrates, proteins, and lipids (fats) that must be broken down to be absorbed into the body and this process is done by enzymes.

Water-soluble or fat soluble

Enzymes are critical in the detoxification process and can either be water-soluble or fat-soluble.

The water-soluble toxins are easily flushed out of the body via the blood and kidneys.

The fat-soluble toxins which include food additives, pesticides, pollutants, preservatives, and even metals, must undergo a chemical shift to be eliminated from the body. When fat-soluble toxic enters the body, the liver converts them into water-soluble substances that can be excreted via watery fluids such as bile or urine.

The elimination process happens mostly in the liver and digestive system. If these are not functioning properly, toxins accumulate in the liver then end up in the blood, fat cells, and brain. They are then stored indefinitely, eventually causing health issues.

Enzymes that are important in detoxification include:

Glucuronidase: This is the key enzyme which adds glucuronic acid to the non-water-soluble substances and converts them to water-soluble forms to be excreted in the urine.

Cytochrome P450: These enzymes are found in the liver and convert fat-soluble into water-soluble for elimination by the kidneys.

Glucuronosyl transferases: These liver enzymes are essential to the disposal of bilirubin, which occurs from the breakdown of red blood cells and is excreted from the body through bile. It also changes other toxins into nonharmful substances by making them more water-soluble.

HOW THE BODY ELIMINATES TOXINS & SALICYLATES

Phenols and Salicylates are metabolised by an enzyme phenol sulfotransferase (PST)

Normally with sufficient levels of sulphates and liver enzymes, phenols are easily metabolised, and the residue is passed out in the urine. Nevertheless, if these enzyme malfunction toxins will build up leading to symptoms.

Phenol sulfotransferase (PST) pathway: PST is a phase 2 liver enzyme that attaches sulphates to phenol compounds to detoxify the body of phenols, salicylates, amines, artificial food, colourings, flavourings, preservatives other toxins. Deficiency, of PST will result in difficulty metabolise certain foods and chemicals that contain phenols and amines. This increases symptoms in salicylate intolerance, a build-up of neurotransmitters in the brain, causing depression, and other mental troubles, and difficulty in the metabolism of adrenaline.

PST enzyme inhibitors: Research suggests Salicylates can suppress the activity of PST enzyme, other inhibitors are food colourants (tartrazine), flavonoids (quercetin).

LIVER DETOXIFICATION PATHWAY *Your liver takes in 3 phases of detoxification*

Phase 1 (breaks down substances) The liver detoxification consists of a group of enzymes known as the cytochrome P450 and are the first line of defence against toxins. They make toxins more water-soluble and into smaller substances that are less harmful. These molecules are transported into your blood and excreted via the kidneys as urine. However, some very toxic end products may remain and must be quickly passed on to phase 2, as with heavy metals, otherwise, they can cause these enzymes to dysfunction.

Phase II (adds on substances) This is the stage that adds on substances to aid detox so that they can be transported easily out of the body. Any toxins from phase 1 will be transformed into water-soluble compounds that can be excreted through urine or bile. This process is done by adding molecules to them (conjugation), and the most important molecules been glutathione (GSH), along with sulphate, and glycine. Normally, at this phase liver enzyme produce low levels of glutathione, but when toxic levels are high, it increases the production of glutathione. *Glutathione:* This is known as the "master antioxidant" and it can rejuvenate itself in the liver, except when the toxic load becomes too large, leading to symptoms. *Antioxidants* are natural or man-made substances that may prevent some types of cell damage and are found in many foods, including fruits and vegetables but is not well absorbed. They act like a magnet drawing free radicals and toxins like lead, mercury, arsenic ready for excretion. Moderate exercise boosts your glutathione levels and helps promote your immune system and improves detoxification.

Phase III This is the transport phase, which requires the excretion of toxins from cells and excreted as urine or bile. Bile is important in moving toxins out of the liver and into the intestines and excreted. Those water-soluble toxins that are gathered in the bloodstream can make their way into the kidneys and excreted through the urine.

Try an Epsom salt bath (magnesium sulphate). Epsom salt is a naturally occurring mineral compound which is readily absorbed through the skin. It is known to remove toxins, as a remedy for several ailments, including reducing swelling. An Epsom salt bath helps restore magnesium and sulphate in your system. Some recommend an Epsom salt bath before bedtime for some fifteen minutes, two to three times per week.

Seek medical advice before using Epsom salts if you are pregnant or suffer any serious complaints.

ENO is an antacid -May help with the excretion of salicylates. This is a fizzy drink made of sodium bicarbonate and citric acid but use with caution as too much can also hasten the excretion of essential nutrients. The effects last about an hour.

Environmental factors

We are always bombarded with chemicals from shops, automobile exhaust, second-hand smoke etc. These toxins can enter your system from the surroundings. Minimise the usage of chemical-based household cleaners and personal wellness care products (cleaners, shampoos, deodorants, and toothpaste), and substitute natural alternatives.

Exercise When possible do at least 30 minutes exercise a day. - anything from running, swimming, dancing. Getting regular exercise is one of the best natural ways to cleanse the body and improves both circulation and digestion.

SOURCE Brandis K. Metabolic Acidosis due to Drugs and Toxins, www.anaesthesiamcq.com/AcidBaseBook/ab8_6c.php. Accessed November 15, 2015. Autism and ADD/ADHD- the PST enzyme. https://www.researchgate.net/profile/Rosemary_Waring. Dr Rosemary Waring (Toxicologists- University of Birmingham UK) She found that most autism spectrum children, are low in sulphate and excrete higher levels of sulphate in urine, due to a deficiency in the PST pathway.

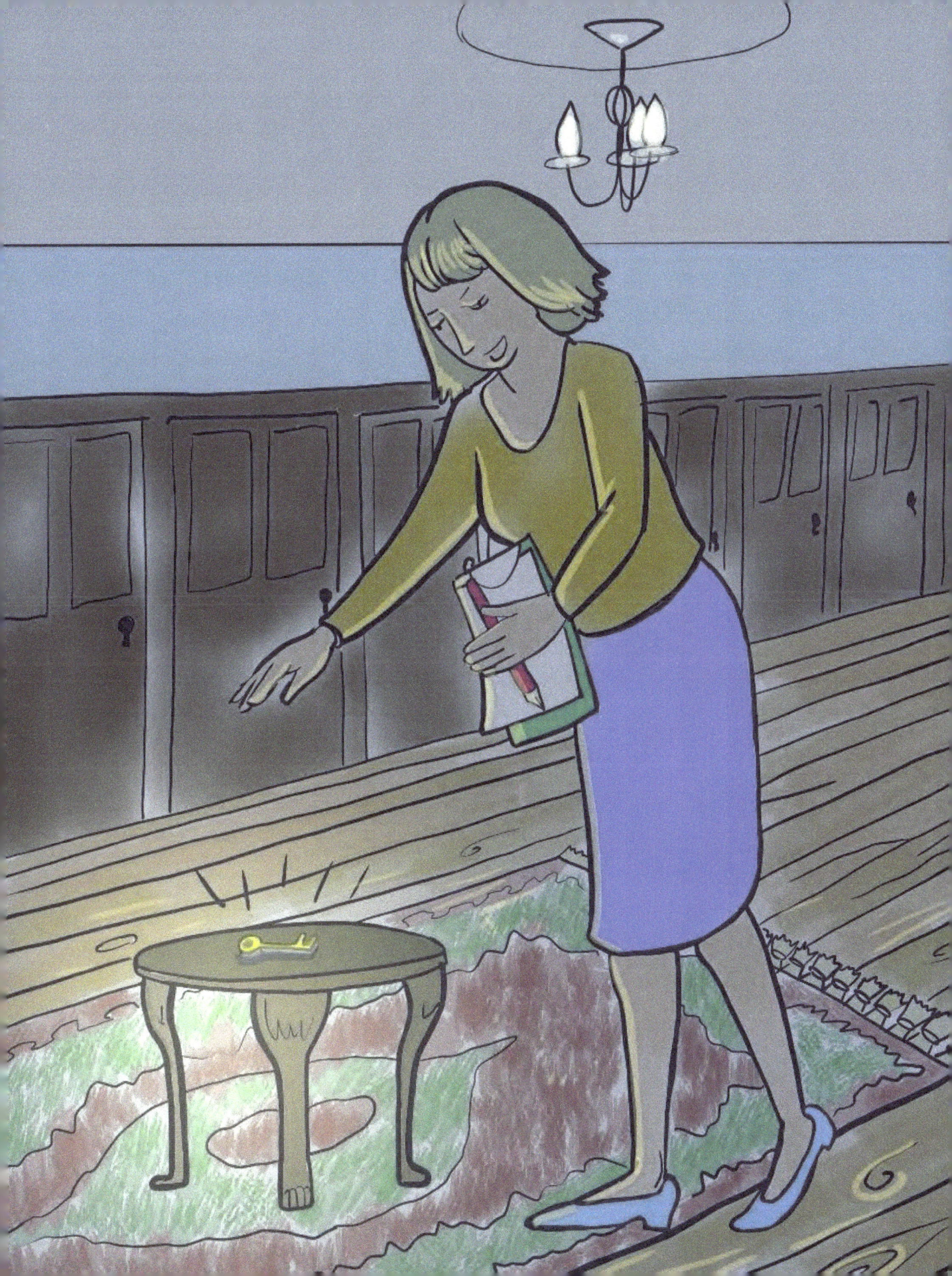

ELIMINATION DIET

Low salicylates

FINDING THE KEY TO HEALTH

Returning to health by removing natural salicylates from your diet

FIRST DISCOVERY OF SALICYLATE IN FOODS

Those with Salicylate Intolerance follow a similar diet as the Feingold diet.

The range of foods that have no salicylate content is very limited, and consequently salicylate-free diets are very restricted.

Dr Feingold a German paediatric allergist was the first to associate dietary salicylates with Intolerance to food when he found that sufficiently high levels could cause behavioural problems in children.

His research in 1973 showed that salicylates, artificial colours, artificial flavours, BHA, and BHT causes hyperactivity in children. He proposes that by eliminating artificial phenols and certain fruits, naturally high in phenol and vegetables, children with allergies and ADHD symptoms significantly improved.

The Feingold Program Elimination Diet.

Avoidance of the following:

Products and foods list containing salicylate.

Artificial food colouring (petrochemical dyes- chemical obtained from petroleum and natural gas)

Short list-FD & C Yellow 5, Tartrazine, E102, FD & C Yellow 6, Sunset Yellow, E 110.D & C Yellow 10, Quinoline Yellow, E104.

Artificial flavours, e.g. Vanillin

Artificial fragrances -most are petrochemical based -toiletries, air fresheners, cleaning supplies, art supplies.

Three petroleum-based antioxidant preservatives BHA-Butylated Hydroxy anisole- E 320, BHT-Butylated Hydroxytoluene- E 131, TBHQ-Tertiary Butylhydroquinone- E 319 Artificial sweeteners -aspartame, acesulfame-K, cyclamates, saccharin, sucralose.

SOURCE: The role of natural salicylates in food intolerance by Ann R Swain.
www.slhd.nsw.gov.au/ rpa/ allergy/ research/ students/ 1988/ anne.html.https:/ / en.wikipedia.org/ wiki/ Salicylate_sensitivity

RESEARCH INTO POSSIBLE REACTIONS

TO SALICYLATE

Salicylate Intolerance -Research into possible causes

Aspirin, which is a salicylate is derived from the willow tree. People were having an adverse reaction to taking Aspirin very soon after it was launched. In 1902 Hirschberg study, suggested Aspirin caused hives (acute urticaria) and that diets that excluded foods containing salicylates and/or additives showed that the symptoms went away on exclusion suggesting that salicylates were the cause.

Modern Research on Salicylate Intolerance

Royal Prince Alfred Hospital - Sydney (RPAH) In 1977 the RPAH started to focus on the possible role of dietary substances in recurrent hives (urticaria) and swelling in the face, tongue, abdomen, or arms and legs (angioedema). By 1980 Dr Anne Swain and team published a novel analysis of salicylate contents in food. They published the salicylate content of 333 foods still used today for dietary salicylate avoidance advice.

They found people with salicylate intolerances show symptoms at very low concentrations, between 35 mg/100mg of salicylate food ingestion (One aspirin is 250mg).

Symptoms: these are like aspirin poisoning: nausea, vomiting, sweating, and tinnitus and other.

Genetics links have also been discovered by these researchers so that food intolerance runs in families but can be triggered or made worse by illness or medication or exposure to environmental chemicals.

SOURCE: Sensitivity to food additives, vaso-active amines and salicylates: a review of the evidence. https://ctajournal.biomedcentral.com/articles/10.1186/s13601-015-0078-3. Salicylate Intolerance (Aspirin)-Hanns-Wolf Baenkler, Prof. Dr Pathophysiology, Clinical Spectrum, Diagnosis and Treatment. Https://www.ncbi.nlm.nih.gov/pmc/articles/PMC2696737/. Salicylate Intolerance (Aspirin) Journal of physiology and pharmacology 2005, http://www.eaaci.org/attachments/9c%20-%20raithelSalicylINT.pdf

SALICYLATE ELIMINATION DIET

It is advisable to seek medical advice before starting an elimination diet

An elimination diet is utilised to distinguish foods that an individual cannot consume without adverse effects. It is a short-term eating plan from two weeks to two months that eliminates certain foods that may be causing adverse reactions.

Low Salicylate Diet for two Weeks (see page chapter on low salicylate diet)

A low salicylate diet is avoiding food that has high levels of salicylates in them and excluding additives or preservatives. By these exclusions, its help to prevent a build-up of toxins from salicylates in your system and should relieve symptoms. You may detect at first that you experience flu like symptoms due to the gradual detoxification of your body from the high levels of salicylates. If you are otherwise unwell the process of elimination of salicylates will be slower.

Starting the diet

Starting a new restricted diet can be very intimidating as it involves some preparation on your part, otherwise you can end up making the same meals. However, to make life more leisurely for you I have included a cookery book which will aid with many varied recipes. Try to stick to the diet strictly for at least two weeks. It is important to keep a food diary to see what you can tolerate, and you may find you can tolerate some moderate levels of salicylates whereas others may only tolerate low salicylates. In the end, once you have five good days in a row without symptoms you can start reintroducing more moderate foods back into your diet. After 4 weeks if the symptoms have not improved it is improbable that you have salicylate intolerance as the effects are likely done by something else but check with your physician or nutritionist.

Balanced Diet: Despite the difficulties in keeping your diet balanced with salicylate Intolerance; there is plenty of nutrient rich foods you can add to your diet.

Start by keeping a food diary

Keeping a food diary will help you gain some insight into what you're eating and how it affects your health and shows what ingredient might be causing the problem.

Write down the date, the time you eat as soon as you can and take note of everything you eat meals, drinks, snacks, biscuits, sweets, no matter how small.

Record how you feel after eating each item. Wait for about 20 minutes after eating to assess how you feel and include any physical symptoms or side effects for example, you might feel nauseous and have an upset stomach.

This trial, error and elimination will help identify suspected food to see if symptoms start out more serious, then the food is reintroduced to ensure whether the symptoms reappear.

PLAN FOOD MENU FOR THE WEEK

I find it makes life easier by planning the menu for the week ahead and I try to cook in batches and freeze the leftovers. This way, on the days you are not feeling well, you already have your food sorted!

Travel For long journeys, I pack a picnic and I usually have some frozen bread rolls ready in the freezer. For long flights take your own snacks and bring enough food to last you for the first few days. For my holidays I always go for self-catering and bring a few tins of salmon and rice in a bag and this gives me a few days to find the shops.

Eating out When eating out it is easier to employ the term allergy because if you say intolerance, they will inevitably think of all the other intolerances and miss the target. I rarely eat out now because you can't expect people to understand and many have failed in the past, with the result that I have, vomited either immediately or several hours later or felt toxic for days afterwards.

I had to laugh once my lovely nieces and daughter in law kindly ordered a completely plain, fresh steak to be cooked simply in butter. They explained a little about my intolerance and showed the waiter my EpiPen to prove a point.

When I had just finished the steak, I found a small pepper corn stuck to my tooth. It wasn't enough to cause a reaction, thankfully, but I've made a point now that when I go out for a meal with the family, I just relax with a soda water, and make sure to eat beforehand instead.

Antihistamines, they're effective in combating reactions, but I personally find it best to only take them when I notice swelling in my face or I am feeling particularly ill. I generally take them at night because the ones I take can make you drowsy.

SOURCE: Royal Prince Albert Hospital Sydney and they are the leading experts on salicylate intolerance The Simplified Elimination Diet booklet introduction https://www.slhd.nsw.gov.au/rpa/allergy/resources/foodintol/handbook.html. The Failsafe Diet http://www.failsafediet.com/the-rpah-elimination-diet-failsafe/

SALICYLATE FREE FOOD OR NEGLIGIBLE -Swain & el

FRUIT

Banana *(A), lime, canned & fresh pear (in sugar syrup) – peeled

VEGETABLES

Potatoes, bamboo shoot, savoy cabbage (green or white), celery, iceberg lettuce, peas, swede.

PULSES

Beans – dried (not borlotti), use canned beans with filtered water preferably. Chick-pea, green split peas and brown lentils.

GRAINS

Barley, buckwheat, millet, oats, rice (white basmati rice), rice cereals (plain) rye, wheat.

SEEDS AND NUTS

Poppy seeds

SWEETENERS

Carob, coca, white sugar, caster sugar icing sugar, brown sugar, glucose, rice malt, syrup, pure maple syrup. However, you should avoid raw sugar such as demerara or muscovado as it is refined sucrose that still has some of its natural molasses.

MEAT

Most meats are safe. Such as: beef, chicken, lamb, offal (organ meats), rabbit, veal. Avoid liver, and processed meats, as they often contain salicylates and nitrates that are used as preservatives and colour fixatives.

Eggs are fine *A = has amines*

As research finds out more about salicylates in foods this list may vary

SEAFOOD

Most fresh plain fish (like salmon, cod, plaice, scallops etc.) are safe, avoid smoked fish and prawns.

HERBS & SPICES

Malt vinegar, saffron, sea salt, soy sauce (if free of added spices).

BAKING

Salt, sodium bicarbonate, citric acid, cream of tartar, gelatine, baker's yeast. Arrowroot, corn flour, golden syrup *(check ingredients some variations)*, malt, malt extract, rice flour, rye flour, sago, soy flour, tapioca, wheat flour, sugar (brown, caster, granulated, icing, powdered).

SEASONING'S

Malt vinegar, saffron, sea salt, soy sauce (if free of added spices).

OILS AND FATS

Butter, cold pressed oils such as sunflower, sunflower, soy, canola oil (crisco), margarine. Always check for preservatives that may mimic salicylate reactions

DAIRY. *Some salicylate sensitive react to milk, may be additives or chemicals or flavourings*

Butter, cream, most plain cheeses (not blue vein) without preservative or additives, yoghurt (plain natural).

Milk (cows or goats), rice, soy milk, ice cream (some have E numbers so watch labels). Tofu.

MISCELLANEOUS Carob powder, cocoa, tofu

BEVERAGES Decaffeinated coffee: check if they use chemicals! The Swiss technique uses only water. Other drinks: Water, Ovaltine, pear juice (homemade), I find Schweppes soda water to be fine. Other makes can be alright be you need to read labels.

ALCOHOL Gin, whiskey, vodka.

CROWS is the easy way to remember which seeds or grains are salicylate-free: corn, rice, rye, oats, wheat, soy.

LOW SALICYLATE IN FOOD

FRUIT

Golden delicious apples (green variety only), papaya *(A) (paw paw), pomegranate (some sources say it's moderate rather than low), nashi pears, tamarillo.

Canned Pear - If these are in sugar syrup, they have negligible amounts of salicylate. However, natural juices/syrups, which often contain the peel will be moderate in salicylates.

VEGETABLES

Brussels sprouts, borlotti beans, cabbage green/red, chickpeas, chives, choko (chayote pear), green beans, green peas, leek, munge bean sprouts, shallots, spring/salad onions, yellow split peas.

NUTS AND SEEDS

Cashews, hazelnuts, pecan, sunflower seeds.

SWEETENERS

Caramel (homemade), golden syrup, malt extract.

SEASONING'S, CONDIMENTS, SAUCES & TOPPINGS

Chives, fennel dried, garlic, soy sauce (if free of spices)

OILS AND FATS

Ghee

Snacks Plain potato chips (read the ingredients list)

BAKING AIDS

Salt, bicarbonate of soda, citric acid, cream of tartar, gelatine, baker's yeast. Baking powder is bicarbonate of soda plus cream of tartar which acts as a raising agent in baking, vanilla extract, vanilla bean. *Vanilla essence is not to be used as it is artificially derived vanillin, which is frequently made from a by-product of the wood pulp.*

BEVERAGES Dandelion coffee also called tea *A = has amines*

MODERATE SALICYLATE IN FOOD

FRUIT

Red golden delicious apples, canned or dried fig, custard apple, lemon, loquat, mango, passion, fruit, persimmon, rhubarb, fresh tomato.

VEGETABLES

Asparagus, tinned, aubergine, beetroot, black olives, carrot, fresh tomato, lettuce (other than iceberg), marrow, mushrooms, parsnips, potato (new and red), pumpkin, snow peas, sweet corn, turnip.

NUTS AND SEEDS

Desiccated coconut, peanut butter, pumpkin seeds, sesame seeds, walnuts.

SWEETENERS

Molasses, raw sugar.

SEASONING'S, CONDIMENTS, SAUCES & TOPPINGS

Fresh coriander leaves (also known as Chinese parsley), horseradish, mayonnaise, parsley.

OILS AND FATS

Almond oil, corn oil, peanut oil.

DAIRY & SOY PRODUCTS

Blue vein cheese.

BAKING

Sesame seeds.

BEVERAGES

Coca cola, rose hip tea, rose hip syrup. ALCOHOL Cider, beer, sherry, brandy.

HIGH SALICYLATE IN FOOD

FRUIT

Apple (but golden delicious is low in salicylates) – all other varieties, canned morello cherries, cantaloupe, grapefruit, kiwi fruit, lychee, mandarin, mulberry, nectarine, peach, watermelon, tomato products.

VEGETABLES

Alfalfa sprouts, artichoke, aubergine with peel, broad bean, broccoli, canned black & green olive, cucumber, eggplant, fresh spinach, okra, radish, sweet potato, water chestnut, watercress, zucchini, capsicum, champignon, chicory, chilli, peppers, courgette, endive, gherkin, peppers, radish, tomato, watercress, zucchini.

NUTS AND SEEDS Brazil nuts, macadamia nuts, pine nuts, pistachio.

SEASONING, CONDIMENTS, SAUCES & TOPPINGS

All spice, bay leaf, caraway, cardamom, cinnamon, cloves, coriander, ginger, mixed herbs, mustard, pimiento.

OILS AND FATS

Copha, sesame oil, walnut oil.

GRAINS Breakfast cereals that include fruit, nuts, honey or coconut corn/maize cereals, cornmeal, flavoured breakfast cereals, maize, polenta

MEATS Fish canned in an unacceptable oil and/or with seasoning's added gravy made from

prepared mixes (stock cubes/bouillon/meat extracts/etc.)

BAKING Corn syrup

BEVERAGES

Regular coffee, all teas, cordials and fruit flavoured drinks, fruit and vegetable juices. ALCOHOL Liquor, port, wine, rum

VERY HIGH SALICYLATE IN FOOD

FRUIT All dried fruits, apricot, avocado, blackberry, blackcurrant, blueberry, cherries.

cranberry, currant, date, grape, guava, loganberry, orange, pineapple, plum, prune, raisin,

raspberry, redcurrant, rock melon, strawberry, sultana, tangerine.

VEGETABLES Fresh olives, capsicum, champignon, chicory, chilli, peppers, courgette, endive, gherkin, radish.

NUTS AND SEEDS

Almond, peanuts with skins on, water chestnut

SEASONING'S, CONDIMENTS, SAUCES & TOPPINGS

Aniseed, basil, black pepper, cayenne, celery powder, chilli flakes, chilli powder, cider vinegar, commercial gravies & sauces, cumin, curry, dill, fenugreek, fish/meat tomato pastes, garam masala, ginger, mace, marmite, mint, mustard, nutmeg, oregano, paprika, peppermint, rosemary, sage, tabasco, tarragon, thyme, turmeric, vegemite and other white pepper, white vinegar, wine vinegar, Worcester sauce.

Yeast Extracts: yeast extract is used sauces, savoury yeast extract spread on their sandwiches, used by food producers to season their products.

OILS AND FATS Coconut oil, olive oil

MEAT Processed luncheon meats (many are seasoned and thus contain salicylates), seasoned meats (e.g. salami, sausages, frankfurters, and hot dogs)

SWEETS Chewing gum with fruit flavours, honey, honey flavours, jam, liquorices, mint flavoured sweets, peppermints.

COMMERCIAL SNACKS Fruit flavoured candy, gelato, sherbet, sorbet, and sweets, liquorice/liquorices (all flavours), mint/peppermint/wintergreen flavoured candy/sweets, pickles (and anything pickled)

BEVERAGES Cordials and fruit flavoured drinks, fruit and vegetable juices, tea.

SHOPPING LIST UK

The ingredients in food are in a constant state of flux so you need to be vigilant.

Salicylates free products are difficult to find because:

Medical research is still ongoing Salicylates are found in many foods, medicines, herbs and botanicals. Personal care products contain salicylates but are not clearly labelled. Companies that say salicylate free products include ingredients such as benzoic acid or colourants. This is a general list but be aware manufactories can change the ingredients so check packets. Also, there many more salicylate free there and with a little research can be found.

List is based on a low-salicylate diet

Vegetable: brussels sprouts, celery, swede, potatoes white, red/green cabbage, iceberg lettuce, spring onions/shallots, leeks, garlic, chives, chokos.

Beans: butter beans, dried lentils beans, kidney beans, munge beans sprouts, bamboo shoots, soy beans, green beans Dried Vegetables: chick peas, lentils, split peas, borlotti beans, soy beans, black eyed beans, cannelloni beans, lima beans, red kidney beans. Tinned Vegetables: green bean, lima beans, butter beans. kidney beans, borlotti beans, chickpeas, beans sprouts, bamboo shoots.

Fruit: bananas, pears bartlett (Williams), packham (not apple shaped), papaw, pomegranates (some lists say low others moderate)

Tinned: Pears in syrup (but not natural juice)

Flour: plain/self-raising, wheat flour (wheaten corn flour), durum wheat semolina flour, soy flour, barley flour.

Pasta: spaghetti, durum wheat, barley rye.

Rice: white, brown plain, rice bran, rice cakes. Brand: -kallo brand rice puffs

Noodles: plain noodles, instant rice noodles

Wheat: couscous, semolina

Bread: Plain white or wholemeal homemade (most shop bought breads have E numbers E280-E283.Crumpets, all butter croissant (check some says butter and have other oils)

Brand-Tortillas Old El Paso, Pita bread newbury phillips organic, wholemeal bread cranks organic,

Please note that in Australia shallots are salad onions in England

Sweeteners: sugar: white sugar, brown sugar light, caster sugar, icing sugar. (avoid sugar made from beets buy only cane sugar). Golden Syrup: Brand-crazy jack organic fair-trade golden syrup. Maple syrup: (source of manganese and zinc). Pure maple syrups are always labelled with a maple leaf logo. Avoid maple-flavoured syrups which contain high fructose corn syrup and small amounts of maple sap. *Note: Tate and Lyle - golden syrup: Some sources say it is high in Salicylate perhaps because it can be made from either inverted sugar syrup or sugar beet juice, sugar beet (beta vulgarise).*

Carob: (high in fibre) comes from carob pods Sweets: white marshmallows Brand-green & black organic chocolate, co-op white chocolate. Topping/caramel syrup: Brand-nestle carnation caramel. Biscuits: shortbread biscuits-all butter biscuits, plain rice cracker. Brand-walkers, Arnott's nice, Ryvita crispbreads, Jacobs cream crackers, Ritz original crackers. Desserts: yoghurt (natural and vanilla), sago and tapioca, Ice creams. Spreads/Jam: golden syrup, malt extract, home-made pear jam only.

Nuts: cashew nuts, pecan nuts (low salicylates), hazelnuts. Flour: plain and self-rising flour, bread flour, check ingredients.

Pasta: all plain pasta, couscous,

Rice: plain rice, medium or long grain but not flavoured like basmati rice.

Salt: sea salt or rock salt

Snacks: brand-kettle crisps

Note: some crisps can have preservatives E 220, 228 or antioxidants if cooked in oils.

Frozen: garden peas, brussels sprouts, swede, savoy cabbage,

butter beans, lima beans. All butter croissants (check labels), all butter scones.

Brand-McCain chips in sunflower oil, pastry - jus-roll all butter puff - pastry, Jus-roll all-butter short - crust.

Beverages: decaffeinated coffee

Note: not all decaf is safe to use because chemicals are used to remove the caffeine. Some use the Swiss method which uses pure water and no chemicals, such as Kenco gold blend, and costa coffee shop are some that use this method.

Milk, soy milk, rice milk, water. soda water, tonic water, homemade pear juice, homemade lemonade. Brand- Ovaltine,

Alcohol: gin, whiskey, vodka

On publishing this list was accurate but manufactures keep changing the recipes!

Cereal grain: wholegrain flaked barley, semolina, porridge oats, rolled oats, puffed rice, millet, amaranth, buckwheat, quinoa cereals.

Brand- Weetabix, bran flakes, rice krispies, Kellogg coco pops, oats so simple(plain), special K, Waitrose rice pops.

Cooking Oils: Sunflower oil, canola oil, safflower oil (avoid synthetic antioxidants 310-321)

Dairy: milk: cow's milk, goats' milk, rice milk - rice dream.

Ice cream: Brand-Kelly of Cornwall clotted cream Ice cream, green and black's vanilla ice cream, Jude Ice cream.

Yoghurt: plain yoghurt, soy yoghurt, cream fraise, fromage frais plain.

Cheeses: most plain cheeses. Brand- Philadelphia

Butters: most butters are fine but avoid spreadable butters as they have additives.

Eggs: fresh eggs

Vanilla: Only use extract or vanilla beans, Brand- Nielsen Massey pure vanilla extract

Meats: preservative free beef, lamb, veal etc.

Poultry: fresh or frozen chicken (no seasoning, self-basting, stuffing).

Seafood: very fresh e.g. cod, whiting, crab, lobster, oysters, calamari, scallops. fresh tuna, salmon, frozen or canned fish including tuna, salmon, or sardines in spring water. No prawns as they contain sulphite preservatives.

Toiletries

Soap: use plain unperfumed

Shampoo: plain, unperfumed, or lightly perfumed shampoo and conditioner.

Toothpaste: Plain, unflavoured.

Moisturisers: organic soya oil (full of vitamin E and non-greasy). Pure shea butter (good for sunburn). Pure vitamin E oil (scars, dry skin, lips). Cocoa butter (good for dry skin).

Emu Oil: The oil helps treat skin infections and other skin conditions.

Cosmetics: Check labels for salicylates and avoid cosmetic or skin preparation which says, "beta hydroxy acid", as this is salicylic acid.

Toilet rolls: plain white rolls as some have additives.

Tissues: plain white only as some have balsam.

Deodorant: Plain unperfumed, bicarb of soda. (See home-made pages), Rock crystal deodorant stick (mineral salts).

Clothes

Dish washing liquid: fairy clear, Palmolive original, earth's friendly dish mate.

Laundry: plain, unperfumed for sensitive skin.

Brands: Surcare, Ecover, Lux, and Amway.

Soap Nuts: these contain real natural soap.

Cleaning Agents: Vinegar, citric acid, bicarb of soda, lye

Microfiber clothes: For general cleaning on their own. (very good)

Vodka - good antiseptic

Note: Milk: craven dale - they pass their milk through ceramic filters to remove the bacteria that turns the milk sour. It's also made without additives or preservatives which is why it's better for you.

Cheese: some chesses contain amines e.g. feta.

Clear Springs- sunflower oil, they also do an unrefined sunflower oil, but this can be quite high in salicylates. Clear springs organic - soy oil, midsummer organic sunflower oil

Toothpaste: although not actually toothpaste these work just as well: baking soda, bentonite clay, activated charcoal powder.

Surcare Non-Biological approved by British allergy foundation. Surcare range of variants do not contain benzoates or Salicylate or enzymes, dyes, acids, or perfumes

Makeup: I use minerals make-up by Lily Lolo made with just 4 ingredients. It also helps protect your skin against the sun UV rays.

Please be aware that there is some company's claiming to be salicylate free products, but they use parabens and sodium benzoates to preserve them.

GETTING ENOUGH FIBRE IN YOUR DIET

A diet rich in fibre can help the digestive system to act better and prevent constipation. Fibre is an excellent natural cleanser as it helps remove toxins, preservatives and other harmful waste materials that have built up in the digestive tract.

Fibre acts like a sponge, absorbing water so you need to drink enough to prevent constipation. The recommended dietary intake of fibre is 30g a day.

Common good sources of fibre are whole wheat, fruit -pears, banana, leafy greens, beans and nuts, lentils, chickpeas in stews, quinoa and brown rice and oats. A small handful of nuts can have up to 3g of fibre.

Well true to my nursing training I had to get the bowels in somewhere

All this list is negligible to low salicylates

All Grains: Plain crackers: Rye Vita, Ryvita Dark Rye Crisp Bread Rye crisp bread (homemade see recipe page…) Plain grains and their flakes Plain rice (all kinds) Oats and oatmeal, plain oat bran

Vegetables source of fibre Bean sprouts Bamboo shoots Brussels sprouts, fresh Cabbage, green, red, fresh Celery, fresh Chayote squash Green beans, fresh Green peas, fresh Leeks, fresh Lettuce Potato, white, peeled, fresh Shallots

Fruit source of fibre Apple, golden delicious Papaya (paw paw), fresh Pear, canned

Pear, fresh*

Pomegranate, fresh

* Psyllium Husk-Psyllium is a form of fibre made from the husks of the Plantago ovata plant's seeds. It sometimes goes by the name ispaghula., a fibre supplement often used to reduce constipation. *

47

FOOD ADDITIVES

Chemical Similarities

Salicylates are chemically similar to many food colourings and flavourings, also, to nitrates /nitrites, benzoates, oxalates and sulphates/sulphites, and are a major component of many food colourings and flavourings.

European Union (EU) legislation.

To regulate additives, each is assigned a unique number, termed as "E numbers".

FOOD ADDITIVES AND SALICYLATES

Some additives are chemically similar and mimic salicylates and may cause a reaction in some individuals may also react to preservatives

In this chapter, we will be discussing food additives such as preservatives, artificial colours and flavourings, as those who are intolerant to natural food chemicals may also react to common food additives. Some of these additives are chemically like salicylates and may cause reactions, especially to benzoates and tartrazine. Those allergic to aspirin would have to avoid them. To date, the mechanism of food additive reactions is not well understood and there are no tests available.

What are food additives used for? All foods have chemicals, either natural or artificial and have different roles, for increasing shelf-life and improving its taste and appearance. They have been round for centuries, such as pickling, salting bacon and used in wines. In the food industry manufacturers must supply info about any additives used in the foods, followed by its name or E number.

Additives are in groups according to their purpose:

Emulsifiers: stabilisers, gelling agents, and thickeners- help oil and water mix

Antioxidants: stop food from reacting with oxygen-preventing food spoiling

Flavour enhancers: used in savoury foods to enhance the existing flavour

Preservatives: chemical that is added to products to prevent decay

Colourings: improve the coloration of food

Sweeteners: a sugar substitute is a food additive (saccharin and aspartame)

These food additives are known to cause adverse reactions in some susceptible people

Nitrates: processed meats are generally high in nitrates and nitrites (causes rash) MSG (mono sodium glutamate): a flavour enhancer (causes headache) Sulphates: food preserver or enhancer used in wines Colourings: especially carmine (red) and annatto (yellow)

Additives to be avoided for salicylate intolerance

Colour: tartrazine E102, sunset yellow E110 Preservatives: (E200-297) Benzoates (E210-219), Sulphites (E220-227), Nitrates (E249-252) Antioxidants: BHA (E320) & BHT (E321).

Food colouring and preservatives may cause angioedema (Facial/ throat swelling) with or without urticaria (rash).

SOURCE: Sensitivity to food additives, vaso-active amines and salicylates: a review of the evidence https://ctajournal.biomedcentral.com/articles/10.1186/s13601-015-0078-3

ADDITIVES *Check labels for the following which use additives as ingredients:*

E100, E152

Anti-foaming agent

Antioxidant

Aroma

Coating agent

Colouring

Consolidant

Emulsifier

Flavour enhancer

Flour treatment agent

Foaming agent

Gelling agent

Humectant

Modified starch

Preservative

Raising agent

Separating agent

Smelting salt

Stabiliser

Sweetener

FOOD PRESERVATIVES

Preservatives (E200-297) In the food industry food is regulated and given E Numbers, some are harmless, but some may cause a reaction. **Some E number that are safe:** *E101 riboflavin (Vitamin B2), E200-203 sorbate derivatives, E260 acetic acid, E280 propionic acid, E300-304 ascorbic acid derivatives (vitamin C), E330-333 citric acids, E412 guar gum and E578 calcium gluconate.*

Chemical name and E-number to avoid:

__E102 (tartrazine),__ E104 (quinoline yellow), E107 (yellow 2g), E110 (sunset yellow)

E120-E219 inclusive (called benzoates)

E122 (azorubine), E123 (amaranth), E124 (ponceau 4R), E127 (erythrosine), E128 (red 2g)

E131 (patent blue), E132 (indigo carmine)

E621, E622 and E623 (called the glutamates)

OTHER E- numbers may cause reaction: *__Sulphites-__ (E220 – E227) Nitrates and Nitrites- (E 249 – E 252). Antioxidants- (BHA and BHT) (E320 – 321)*

Preservatives in Medical procedures

Dentist: For a local anaesthetic, plain lignocaine should be alright for tooth extraction, but your Dentist can check the ingredients first.

General anaesthetics: Before having an operation, you will meet up with an anaesthetist. He will check with you about your medical history and ask if you have any allergies, for example, to drugs or foods. You can then discuss with the Doctor about your salicylate intolerance and preservatives in some medicines.

Other: Preservative in bread: calcium propionate or mycoban (E282) is a natural acid that works as an antimicrobial preservative in food products, especially in bakery. A couple of slices a day is alright, but I find it best to make my own bread.

Both BHA and BHT were used in the rubber and petroleum industry and they can trigger asthma, allergic rhinitis and urticaria.

FLAVOUR ENCHANCER

Flavour enhancers are labelled with E numbers from E600 to E699 and are used in savoury foods to bring out the existing flavour. For example, mono sodium glutamate is added in processed foods, especially soups, sauces, and sausages.

List of Flavour Enhancer with E numbers

Glutamates and glutamate boosters are frequently hidden as yeast extract, hydrolysed

Vegetable protein HVP or hydrolysed plant protein HPP.

Avoid the following: Glutamates 620 L -glutamic acid 621 Mono sodium L-glutamate or MSG 622 Mono potassium L- glutamate 623 Calcium glutamate 624 Mono ammonium L-glutamate 625 Magnesium glutamate Other flavour enhancers 627 Disodium guanylates 631 Disodium inosinate 635 Disodium ribonucleotides

Allowed: Other flavour enhancers 636 Maltol 637 Ethyl maltol 640 Glycine 641 L-Leucine

Monosodium Glutamate (MSG)

This a food additive and flavour enhancer commonly added to Chinese food, tinned veggies, soups and processed meats. Some people experience mild flushing of the skin and headaches when they eat glutamates or MSG.

What is the difference between Yeast and Yeast extract?

Baker's yeast: this is a fungus that requires sugar to rise and this assists the bread to develop. Yeast Extract: is made from deactivating the yeast itself and used as additives to foods or flavourings that function similarly as MSG or monosodium glutamate. They are added in the cheese, canned soups, stews, frozen dinners, and salty snacks, marmite. *With Salicylate intolerance yeast extract needs to be avoided*

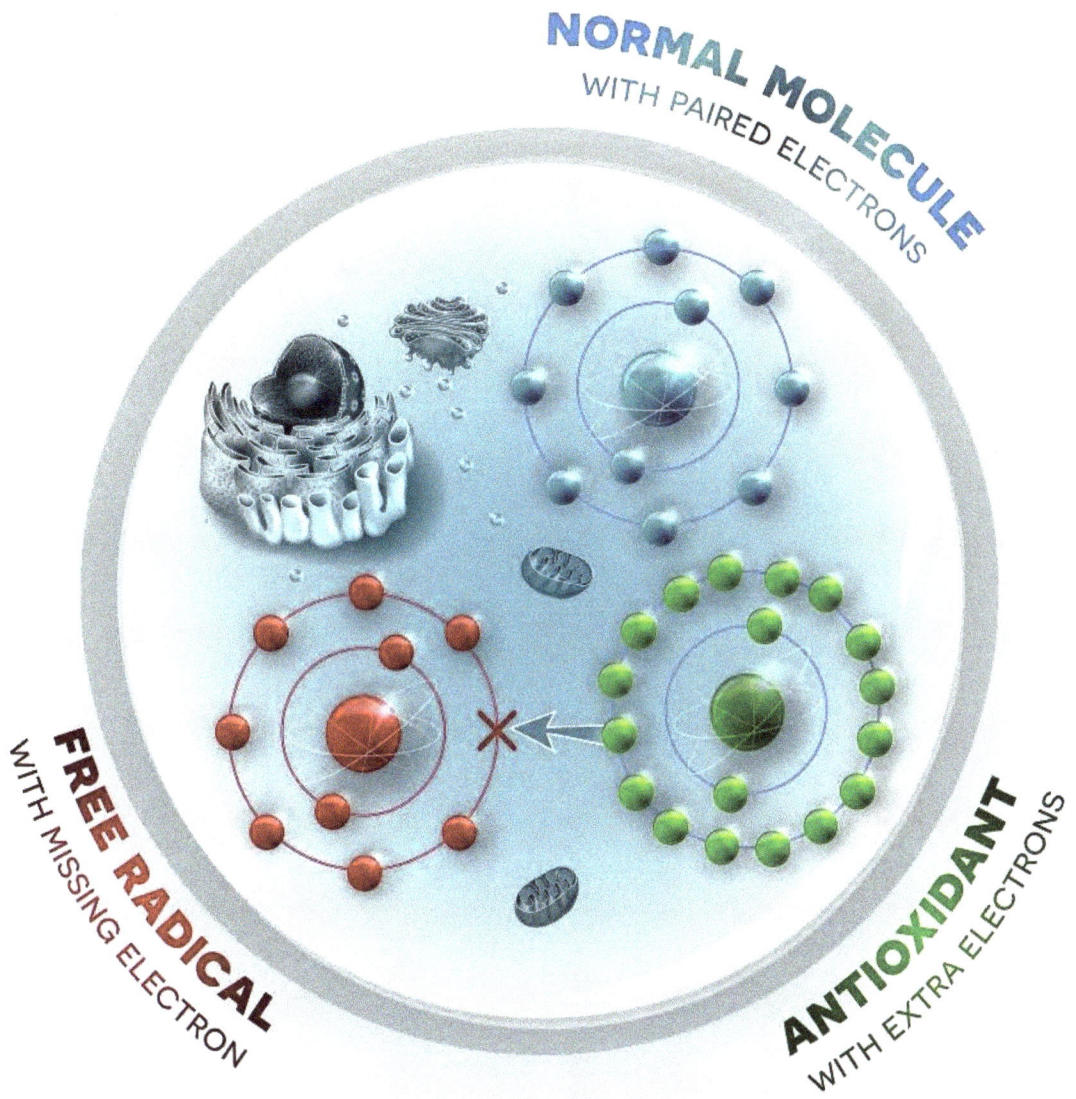

NORMAL MOLECULE
WITH PAIRED ELECTRONS

FREE RADICAL
WITH MISSING ELECTRON

ANTIOXIDANT
WITH EXTRA ELECTRONS

ANTIOXIDANTS

Any flavours with salicylates at the end are not safe to take, for example -benzyl salicylate (raspberry flavour).

What are they? Antioxidants are natural or man-made substances that are used to prevent or delay some types of cell damage from free radicals. Free radicals are molecules that hold single or more unpaired electrons caused for example by smoking. We all have both antioxidants and free radicals present in our systems with some made by the body and others from our diets. Natural-Antioxidants: Some good sources are fruits, vegetables, chocolate, tea, wine, coffee, pecan nuts. There are several nutrients in food that contain antioxidants, vitamin C, vitamin E, and beta carotene are among the most common.

Antioxidants- best avoided:

Man-made- antioxidants (301-321)

Phenol derivatives- BHA, BHT, TBHQ and propyl gallate.

Synthetic antioxidants in the food industry are:

BHA-Butylated hydroxy anisole (E320): found in vegetable oil, spreadable butter

BHT-Butylated hydroxytoluene (E321): most popular synthetic antioxidant food additive TBHQ-Tert-Butylhydroquinone (E319): unsaturated vegetable oils

PG -Propyl gallate (E310) used in oils and fats

The above also found in food packaging, cosmetics, pharmaceuticals, oil products, rubber, hair products, adhesives, lubricants and so on.

Food Flavours are additives that give food a special taste or smell and may be derived from natural ingredients or created artificially.

Here are the different types of flavours added to nutrient:

Natural flavourings: these are natural sources created from anything that is eatable.

Man-made flavours: These are elements that are not edible (petroleum) and maybe artificial versions of precisely the same chemicals that are found in nature, such as vanilla.

Manufacturer can write 'flavour' or 'flavouring' and as a purchaser, you will not recognize if the food is natural or contrived. For example, artificial vanilla is not derived from vanilla beans, but made either from Guayaquil or lining a by-product of the wood pulp industry!

FOOD COLOURING & ADDITIVES

Salicylate intolerant should avoid colourings as these are similar chemically and use the same detox pathway. Natural food colours can be high in salicylates, amines and glutamates

Food colourings or dyes are used pretty much for the role you'd anticipate, to give food and drink a more appetizing appearance. They are also employed in a non-food such as cosmetics and medications. In recent years there have been claims that artificial dyes can cause hyperactivity in children, as well as cancer and allergies but these studies are ongoing.

Some natural colourings Natural food colours originate from a wide range of sources like vegetables, fruits, plants, minerals and other edible natural sources.

Here are just a few examples Caramel colour: this makes cola brown and beer gold. Annatto extract (carotenoid): this is an orange-red food colouring derived from the sources of the achiote tree, often added to the cheese. Cochineal extract (carmine): This is a crimson dye produced from crushed cochineal beetle.

Artificial colours in food These are fabricated by chemical reaction and are normally employed in food and pharmaceutical industries. Some of the common food colours are tartrazine, sunset yellow, amaranth, Allura red, quinoline yellow, bright blue and indigo carmine.

Salicylate Intolerance should avoid the colourings: (E100-180) especially tartrazine E102, sunset yellow E110 as these are similar chemically and use the same detox pathway.

Sunset Yellow(E110): this is a is a petroleum-derived orange azo dye and used in food, cosmetics, and drugs. (banned in some countries).

Tartrazine (E102): The azo dyes tartrazine is primarily utilized as a food colouring with a similar chemical structure to salicylates, benzoates, other azo compounds. It was originally distilled from coal tar and used as a dye for wool and silk, they are by-products of the oil industry.

Foods with tartrazine. Tartrazine is in commercial foods that hold an artificial yellow or greenish coloration.

The following is a list of foods that may contain tartrazine: fruit squash, cordial, coloured fizzy drinks, instant puddings, cake mixes, custard powder, soups, sauces, ice cream, cereals, beverages, sweets, ice creams, jams.

Personal care: conditioners, cosmetics, liquid soaps, lotions, hand sanitizer, perfumes, nail polish, and shampoos.

Medications: Used to give yellow, orange or green hue to a liquid, found in capsule, pill, lotion, or gel, vitamins, antacids, cough syrups and lotions. Household: Tartrazine is also used in other products such as inks, crayons, stamp dyes and glues.

ARTIFICIAL PRESERVATIVES & COLOURINGS

Those who are hypersensitive to aspirin and are salicylate intolerant react to the azo dye tartrazine, and benzoates and sulphites.

Benzoates, Tartrazine, Sulphites

Those who are salicylate intolerant and allergic to aspirin may react to the artificial food colourings and preservatives, called azo dye tartrazine, benzoates, and sulphites. Both salicylic acid and benzoic acid have a similar chemical.

Benzoates are the salt or ester of benzoic acid and are frequently used as pharmaceutical or food preservatives. Benzoic acid occurs naturally in many plants in high concentrations, especially certain berries.

Manufactured Benzoic acid/ food additive Benzoates E numbers are as follows: Benzoic acid (E210), sodium benzoates (E211): the sodium salt of benzoic, potassium benzoate (E212): the potassium salt of benzoic acid, calcium benzoate (E 213), ethyl 4-hydroxy benzoate (E214)

Products with Benzoic acid Benzoic acid inhibits the growth of mould, yeast and some bacteria and they are used in processed foods such as meats.

Here is a list of that may have benzoic acid as an element

Food: some yoghurt, cheeses, chocolates, ice creams, pickles, desserts, pickles, spicy sauces, ready meals, kidney beans, broccoli, spinach, tea, beer and so on

Cosmetics: many cosmetics use benzoic acid to prevent infections caused by bacteria. Body care, mouthwashes, deodorants, toothpaste, aftershave lotions and sunscreens, face washes, creams, and make-up

Medical Skin Care: some products use them to help treat skin irritation and inflammation caused by burns, insect bites, eczema, and fungal infections such as ringworm.

Side effects of benzoic acid: These include gastrointestinal irritation, asthma, rashes and itching and irritation of your skin and eyes, urticaria, angioedema.

Parabens hypersensitive are chemical compounds based on Para hydroxybenzoic acid and act as preservatives. These chemicals are typically found in cosmetics, but they may also appear in food items and health care aids. Common parabens include: methylparaben (E218), ethyl paraben (E214), propylparaben (E216), butylparaben and heptyl paraben (E209).

SOURCE: Benzoic acid and sodium benzoate https://www.who.int/ipcs/publications/cicad/cicad26_rev_1.pdf. Major study suggests a link between hyperactivity in children and certain food additives https://www.southampton.ac.uk/news/2007/09/hyperactivity-in-children-and-food-additives.page.The University of Southampton and Imperial College London carried out this research. the medical journal, The Lancet. We now have clear evidence that mixtures of certain food colours and benzoate preservative can adversely influence the behaviour of children. Sensitivity to food additives, vase-active amines, and salicylates: a review of the evidence https://www.ncbi.nlm.nih.gov/pmc/articles/PMC4604636/

NITRATES & NITRITES MINERALS

Salicylates are very similar in chemical structure to nitrates and nitrites and although rare, people with Salicylate Intolerance react to them with food.

What are Nitrates? Nitrates are a naturally occurring mineral, which is formed as part of the natural breakdown of organic matter. Anything that grows from the ground draws sodium nitrate out of the soil so that levels are lower in fruits compared to vegetables because the further the fruit is away from the nitrate-rich soil, the lower the concentration of nitrate in its flesh and seeds. For instance, apples were found to have only trace quantities of nitrates. Sodium nitrate is present in many vegetables such as carrots, celery, and many fruits and cereals. Nitrate is particularly effective as a food preservative. In industry, nitrates are manufactured as fertilisers, dyes and even explosives. They are used in medicine because they cause the blood vessels to widen and help treat chest pain associated with angina and reduce the symptoms of congestive heart failure. **Allergies to Nitrates**.

Some people may be allergic to nitrates and react after ingestion of processed meats containing nitrate or nitrite salts. They may suffer from headache, diarrhoea, or urticaria after ingesting them and it can contribute to life-threatening condition – anaphylaxis.

What are Nitrites? Nitrites are naturally occurring minerals, formed by soil microorganisms that break down animal matter. They are used as a food preservative for colouring and flavouring meat (such as ham and bacon) and fish products. Broadly speaking, the combination of sodium nitrates, benzoates, and sulphites are more likely to set off an allergic response than one single food preservative. Avoiding processed meats is a safe path to cut down your intake of nitrates and nitrites

What is the difference between Nitrates and Nitrites? The main difference is that nitrate contains one nitrogen atom and three oxygen atoms, whereas nitrite group contains one nitrogen atom and two oxygen atoms. The term nitrites are often used interchangeably with nitrates, due to the conversion in the body of nitrate to nitrite.

Conversion of nitrate to nitrites -known as the entero-salivary circulation. The digestive system converts nitrate consumed through fruits, vegetables, and grains into nitrite. Nitrates and nitrites circulate from the digestive system, into the blood, then into the salivary glands and part of it is converted by mouth bacteria into nitrite and then back into the digestive. They are disposed of by the body via the urine system. This procedure is necessary to help maintain the digestive system healthy by killing of microorganisms, such as salmonella.

Ways to reduce Nitrites & Nitrates in foods

Nitrates are relatively harmless until they are converted into nitrites. Major food companies put the preservatives nitrates and nitrites, into such food as sandwich meats, bacon, salami, or sausages to give them colour and to extend their shelf lives.

Avoiding processed meats Check ingredients and avoid sodium or potassium nitrates and nitrites in canned beans and vegetables with bacon, and packaged seafood. Use organic foods when possible as these don't have preservatives. Bacon joints- Boil bacon a couple of times and skim off nitrates that come to the surface.

Nitrosamines

Nitrosamines are compounds produced when nitrite, combines with amino acids in the stomach. Research has shown nitrosamines are implicated in cancers of the stomach, oesophagus, nasopharynx, and urinary bladder. By law, producers must restrict the number of nitrites they use in processed meats, because of the dangers of nitrosamines.

E numbers ("E" stands for "Europe") are codes for substances used as food additives. Here are the number for Nitrates and Nitrites- E 252, E251, E249, E250, the combination of sodium nitrates, benzoates, and sulphites may cause an allergic response than one single food preservative.

SOURCE: Nitrate and beetroot juice supplementation reduce blood pressure in adults,
https://www.ncbi.nlm.nih.gov/pubmed/23596162.https://academic.oup.com/ajcn/article/90/1/11/4596779. Nitrosamine and oesophageal cancer risk,
https://ecnis.openrepository.com/handle/10146/25215. https://journals.plos.org/plosone/article?id=10.1371/journal.pone.0119712

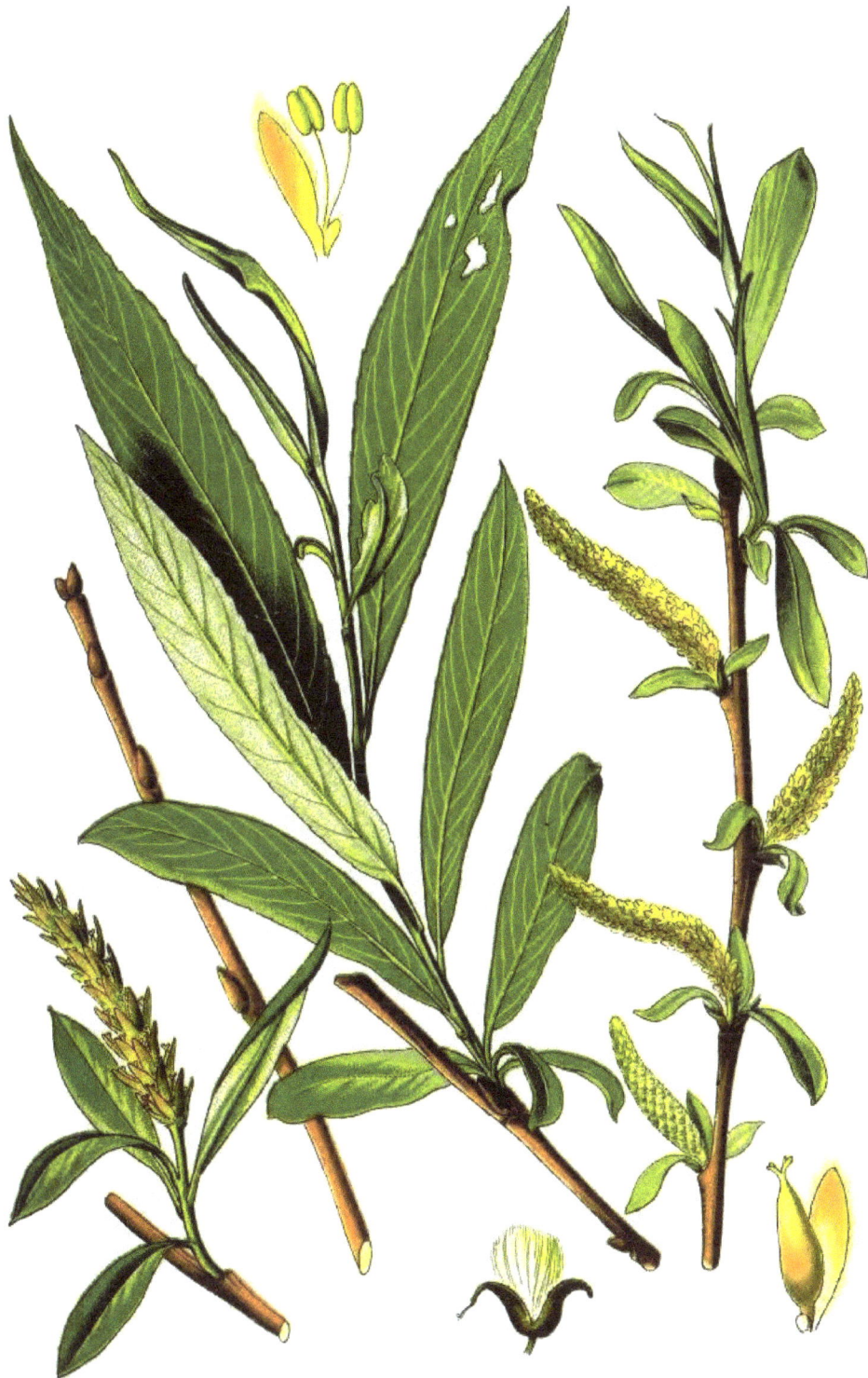

Salix alba

White willow (Salix alba) is a natural source of salicylic acid

SULPHUR

Which cause reactions

Salicylate intolerant react to Sulphites, Tartrazine, Benzoates

Research suggest that 5% of people with Salicylate intolerance & Aspirin allergies also, suffer from Sulphite allergies or Sulphite intolerance

SULPHUR- ESSENTIAL FOR DETOXIFICATION

Sulphur is crucial for detoxification and are essential to detox Salicylate. Salicylate intolerant may react to Sulphites

SULPHUR & SULPHITES

Sulphur plays a key role in detoxification and people who struggle with toxicity will often have a deficiency.

Sulphur is the third most abundant mineral in the body and is present in all living tissues. It is

major component of two essential amino acids: cysteine and methionine, which are important for metabolism and regulating the body's insulin. It boosts the immune system, helps maintain healthy joints and contributes to fat digestion and absorption.

Sulphur in food Sulphur is a naturally occurring compound found in protein-rich foods and certain vegetables. Some good sources of dietary sulphur are eggs, garlic, meat, poultry, fish, milk, shallots, garlic, leek, cabbage, brussels' sprouts, celery, nuts, cashews.

Causes of Sulphur deficiency anaphylaxis. occurs when nutrients are grown in sulphur-depleted land. It can likewise ensue from eating low-protein diets and a deficiency of intestinal bacteria which are essential for metabolism.

Sulphur deficiency can contribute to: Pain and inflammation associated with various muscle and skeletal disorders.

Enzymes cannot function properly, leading to health issues. May contribute to a toxic build-up as in various food intolerance including salicylate Intolerance.

SOURCE: Are you getting enough sulphur in your diet? https://www.researchgate.net/publication/5861075_Are_we_getting_enough_sulfur_in_our_diet. EpiPen: This injection for anaphylaxis contains sodium metabisulphite, but the presence of a sulphite in this product should not deter administration of the drug for treatment of serious allergic or other emergency situations. Oral challenges to detect aspirin and sulfite sensitivity in asthma. Sulphation Benefits-http://www.epsomsaltcouncil.org/wp-content/uploads/2015/10/sulfation_benefits.pdf web.archive.org/web/20081120081902/http://www.aaaai.org/aadmc/ate/sulfites.html

Manufactured Sulphur are produced from oil and gas and is known as elemental sulphur. They are used in fertilisers, chemicals, medicine, sugar, detergents, plastics, and paper. In medicine Sulphonamides (non-antibiotic) has anti-inflammatory properties, reduces pain and swelling of arthritis.

Magnesium sulphate is used as a laxative. Epsom salt bath increase sulphur levels.

Methionine Homocysteine Cysteine Cystine Taurine -amino acids

Methionine: This produces cysteine and taurine, which is essential for detoxifying processes, and for growth of connective tissue, such as blood vessels, bone, hair.

A deficiency can lead to inflammation of the liver and it is used to prevent liver damage in Tylenol poisoning. Methionine is found in protein such as meat, fish, and dairy.

Homocysteine: Protein foods containing methionine are transformed into homocysteine in the bloodstream and then converted in the body to cysteine, with the aid of vitamin B6. Homocysteine can also be recycled back into methionine using vitamin B12-related enzymes. An abnormal accumulation of homocysteine indicates heart disease.

Cysteine: This produces taurine and the antioxidant glutathione which is crucial for detoxification in the liver. As an amino acid it is a component of skin (elasticity) causes keratin to be very hard and is present in all high-protein foods.

Cystine: This is constituted from two cysteine molecules linked together. Methionine is needed in the diet, to produce cystine and to prevent deficiency. Cystine also helps make glutathione, keratin, vitamin B6, and insulin.

Taurine: This is derived from cysteine and methionine and occurs naturally in the human brain. It is thought to have antioxidant properties and help congestive heart failure (CHF).

Cysteine and Cystine? Cysteine is formed from homocysteine, which comes from methionine whereas cystine is formed when two molecules of cysteine combine, and the process of oxidation takes place.

SULPHITES

Sulphites are also used in food packaging like cellophane

Sulphites (Sulfite)(toxic) Sulphites, or sulphur dioxide are found naturally in some foods and is used as a preservative in wines and foods due to its antibacterial and antioxidant properties. Very rarely, some people suffer allergic responses to them that can run from mild to severe.

Sulphites in our bodies

From amino acids we make sulphite

From sulphite we make homocysteine

From homocysteine we make cysteine

From cysteine we make sulphites

From sulphites we make sulphates

Sulphate(non-toxic) They are derived from sulphite and are needed for making stomach acid and digestive enzymes, so that we can break down the food we eat into useful components. Sulphate are anti-inflammatory and anti-depressant.

Sulphates are manufactured into cleansing agents, and you can find them in anything from your shampoo as sodium laureth sulphate and toothpaste to car wash soaps.

Sulphate detoxification: Without normal levels of Sulphate in the body sulfotransferase enzyme cannot metabolise salicylates, phenols, and other toxins. Sulphides (Sulfides):(E220 – E227) (toxic) These occur in all rock types such as in pyrite, zinc, mercury, copper, silver, and platinum. The primary use for sulphide is in the production of sulphuric acid used for fertilisers.

SOURCE: Sulfate and Sulfation.Sufferers of asthma, allergic rhinitis, aspirin allergies are at an elevated danger of reaction to sulphites http://www.epsomsaltcouncil.org/wp-content/uploads/2015/10/sulfation_benefits.pdf.Depression management https://www.ncbi.nlm.nih.gov/pubmed/25933976

SULPHITING AGENTS

If you are sensitive to sulphites you are not necessarily sensitive to sulphates (and vice versa.) but usually people react to both sulphites and sulphates.

Sulphiting agent are food preservatives which are used to stop spoilage and discolouration of foods served in public places, or are added to packaged foods (e.g., canned seafood, grapefruit juice, beer, and wines).

Here is a list of sulphur derivatives additives and their E numbers

E150b Caustic sulphite, caramel food colouring

E150d Sulphite ammonia, caramel food colouring

E220 Sulphur dioxide-produced commercially, used in agriculture and in the food and beverage industries as, among other things, and a preservative.

E221 Sodium sulphite. It is a product of sulphur dioxide used as a preservative for fruit and for preserving meats.

E223 Sodium metabisulphite

E224 Potassium metabisulphite. It is used in wine and beer as an antioxidant additive.

E226 Calcium sulphite, bleaching agent in sugar production.

E227 Calcium hydrogen sulphite is an antioxidant, preservative (banned in Australia).

E228 Potassium bisulphite made from sulphur dioxide, used for alcoholic beverages.

HISTAMINE & AMINE

Intolerance

Histamines are often the cause of inflammation that results from Salicylates Intolerance

AMINO ACIDS

Salicylate intolerant may develop an amine intolerance

Salicylate Intolerance and Amines

While there is not sufficient evidence for it, some studies suggest that in rare cases, some people who are salicylate intolerant may also develop an Amine Intolerance causing similar symptoms.

What are Amino Acids?

Amino acids are compounds that combine to make proteins which are essential for all living life. The protein ingested from our diet is broken down by enzymes into amino acids, from them the body makes its proteins.

They are essential for the formation of cells, hormones, enzymes, neurotransmitters, and antibodies.

If enough just one essential amino acid is not obtained from food, the body takes that amino acid from muscle tissue and other sources of protein within the body.

Other important Amines

BIOGENIC AMINES

Biogenic amines are one or more amine groups.

There are five well established biogenic amine neurotransmitters: adrenaline (epinephrine), noradrenaline (norepinephrine), dopamine, serotonin, and histamine.

AMINE INTOLERANCE

/HISTAMINE INTOLERANCE

This condition is thought to be related to high levels of histamine that exceeds what is required and therefore accumulate in the body causing symptoms.

However, certain enzymes help break down excess histamine in your body, such as a digestive enzyme (diamine oxidase) and monoamine oxidase (MAO) which cleans up neurotransmitters in your brain. If levels of these enzymes are low, symptoms of intolerance develop.

Symptoms

The symptoms can be triggered by certain foods such as mature cheeses, wine, fermented meats, yeast, fish, chocolate, additives etc.

Diagnosis and treatment of Amines Intolerance are made through dietary exclusion. Some suggest treatment with Diamine oxidase supplement.

Allergies from Histamines

Histamine is a biogenic amine and is released in response to an allergic reaction, virus, or bacterial infection. It can trigger allergic conditions, including hay fever, eczema, asthma, and urticaria.

Antihistamine medications help to fight symptoms caused by the discharge of histamine during an allergic response.

Histamine toxicity or scombroid poisoning: This is sometimes confused with an allergic reaction to fish that contain naturally high levels of the histidine which can be converted to histamine by bacteria. Can cause an allergic response.

Note: In medicine monoamine oxidase inhibitors (MAOI) drugs are used as anti-depressants.

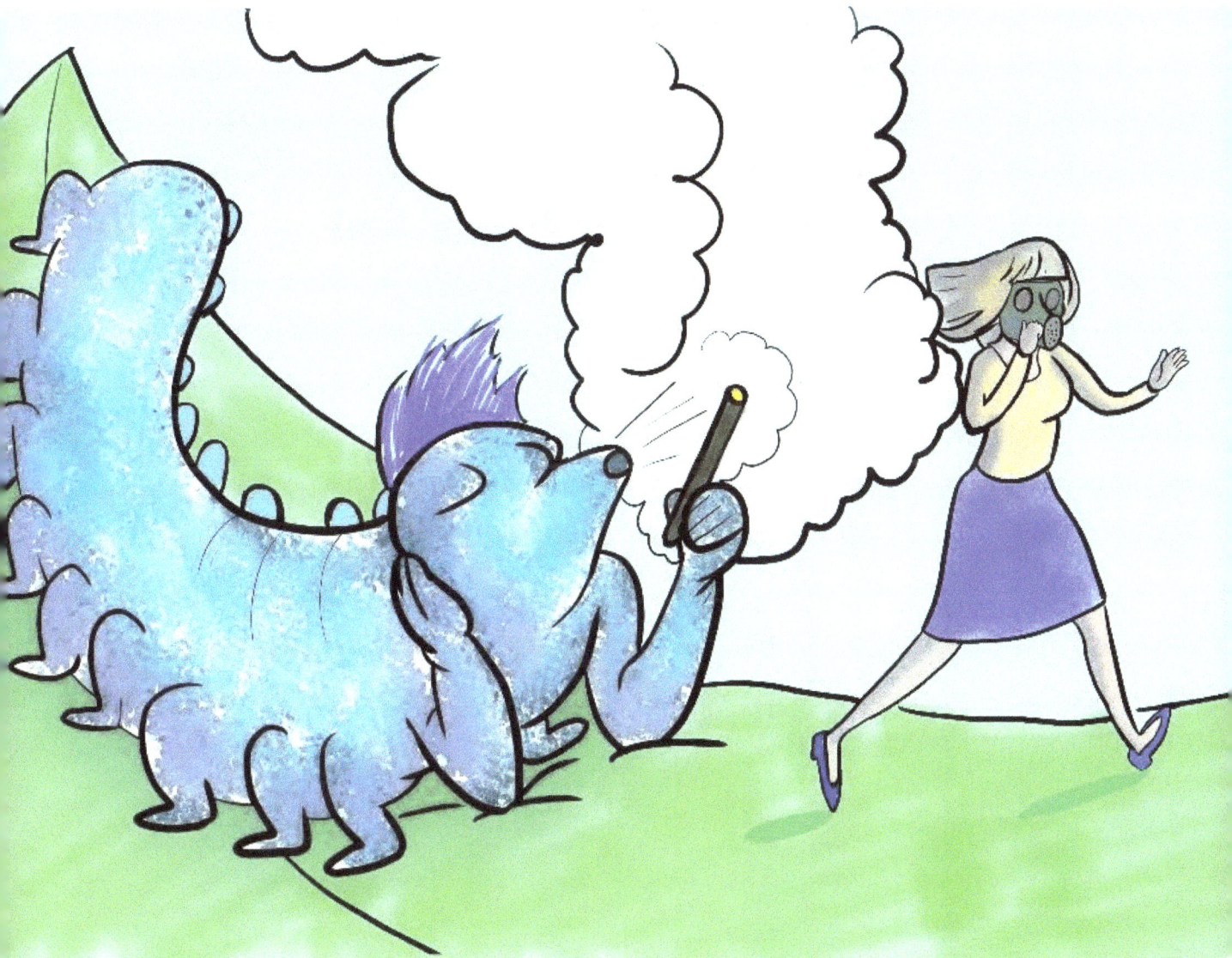

XENOBIOTICS

&

VOLATILE ORGANIC COMPOUNDS

SALICYLATE IN THE ENVIRONMENT

I have had a few Angioedema reactions from chemicals in the environment

Salicylates are in all sorts of places, not just food, and these sources can lead to reactions that are just as severe. Some chemicals in the environment mimic salicylates such as, medications, perfumes, industrial chemicals, plastics, and some pesticides.

Inhaling Smells & fumes

People with salicylate food intolerances may be affected by the scents of flowers, perfumes, essential oils and incense, petrol stations and many more but once you leave the vicinity symptoms usually clear.

Aromatherapy: Essential oils have salicylate in them, for example, methyl salicylate - oil of wintergreen. These are used in many therapies and are best avoided as they may cause a reaction.

Painting & decoration have solvents

Painting and decorating can be a problem, especially as it can take up to a month for even emulsion to cure and dry which can leave a smell. Some products to be aware of oil-based paints, glues, floor varnish, treated wood which can emit volatile chemicals for some time after use.

Chlorine in swimming pools

You may or may not react to chlorine in the water and there is not a lot of research to go by. Nevertheless, be aware that chlorine is processed by the same detox pathway (sulfation pathway) as salicylates. (Consider the chapter on detoxing).

Here are a few hints for protecting yourself when swimming:

Shower immediately before and after swimming using a natural chemical-free soap.

Drink plenty of water before and after you swim to keep hydrated.

Wear goggles to protect your eyes.

Wear a nose plug and keep your mouth closed while swimming.

Be aware that a very strong smell of chlorine means it has too much chlorine.

If possible, try to limit your time in the indoor pool area to just swimming as there are more chemical vapours in the air. Afterwards: Consider having an Epsom salt bath later or an Epsom foot soak to help replace sulphur and aid detox process.

Household things to avoid

During a lot of our household day to day chores, we can be exposed to salicylates, without realising. The best path ahead would be to try and to reduce household cleaners, and instead use vinegar and sodium bicarbonate to clean, which from my experience is 100% safe to use.

Here is a list to help you reduce the contact of environmental salicylates and related.

Laundry: When washing clothes, it is best to avoid perfumed washing powders, fabric conditioners and ironing sprays etc.

New textiles: most textiles have a residue of chemicals used during the manufacturing process, so it is advisable to wash all new textiles before use especially if you will have skin contact.

New Merchandise: These come in at the various seasons and you may have noticed a higher smell in the shops. This is due to the manufacturing process which will soon dissipate.

Gardening: When you are in contact with garden pesticides and weed killers' solutions it would be best to wear gloves to prevent absorption through the skin.

Flooring: new carpets may still have chemicals from the factory and emit them for a few days, so if possible open out in the fresh air before fitting. Wooden flooring may use adhesives which may cause you to have symptoms.

How to reduce the effects of fumes and smells and salicylates in the environment

If you are in an environment where there are high levels of smells you may notice you begin to go a bit nauseated, faint and develop a headache especially in shopping malls. I have often had to exit shops because of the smells and a few times when I was shopping in the household chemical isle.

Usually, you will start to feel better once you go outside for fresh air. It is a good idea to carry a mask for these times or a silk handkerchief.

When you are at home open windows and doors daily to disperse the build-up of smells. When going to hotels ask them to open windows before you come and not to use air fresheners or plugins.

Please note that except for sulphur dioxide and sulphite, a declaration is not required for some additives made of combined substances.

SALICYLATE INTOLERANCE & XENOBIOTICS & VOCs

Those with Salicylate Intolerance may react to chemicals in the environment

Due to chemicals in the environment, I have had a several reactions (angioedema) especially at shopping Mall.

XENOBIOTICS means 'foreign to life' in which chemicals that is not naturally produced or expected to be present within the organism. It has been estimated that humans are exposed to 1-3 million xenobiotics in their lives.

Ingestion of Xenobiotics The major source of xenobiotics in food are additives such as colourings, flavourings, preservatives, antibiotics and industrial chemicals and environmental chemicals.

Natural compounds can also become xenobiotics if they are taken up by another organism, an example of this is the effect experienced by fish that live downstream from the outlet of a sewage treatment plant. Hormones produced by humans may be present, even in treated water and these compounds are foreign to the fish.

When xenobiotics get into your body – usually through contaminated food, water, and air – they can cause serious medical problems such as endocrine disorders, liver toxicity, a suppressed immune system etc.

Still, the good news is that our bodies with the aid of calcium-gluconate and enzymes can detoxify our bodies from Xenobiotics into safer forms, so they don't damage vital organs like the kidneys when excreted. This work is mainly done by the liver and then excreted through urine, bile, faeces, breath, and sweat.

Some ways to avoid Xenobiotics Reduce food additives. Wash fruit and vegetables: before eating, as they might be contaminated with pesticides and pathogenic micro-organisms.

Reduce plastics: and use glass containers for food., because plastics contain Xenobiotics- phenol A (BPA), phthalates. Get rid of as many chemical-based household cleaners, laundry products and air fresheners.

SOURCE: Xenobiotic metabolism- A view through metabolometer, https://www.ncbi.nlm.nih.gov/pmc/articles/PMC2872059/

VOLATILE ORGANIC COMPOUNDS or VOCs

Airborne VOCs These are airborne solvents found both indoor and outside air.

VOCs are both natural and manufactured chemical emitted into the air from products or processes and found in both indoor and outdoor air. Most scents or odours are of VOCs. They are found in gases from burning fuel such as gasoline, wood, coal, and they can act with other gases and form other air pollutants after they are in the air.

VOCs concentrations are normally low, and as such, our bodies generally eliminate them quite efficiently. In some instances, however, VOC's may accumulate, irritating the eyes, nose, and throat, which can cause difficulty breathing and nausea.

Many VOCs are harmful to the environment and human health (e.g. certain paints or petrol) and, as such, are strictly regulated in the UK.

VOCs found in the air indoors and outside.

Concentrations of many VOCs are consistently higher indoors (up to ten times higher) than outdoors.

Indoor VOCs: these are found in smoking, house merchandise, building materials, furnishings, paints, aerosol sprays, varnishes, disinfectants, cosmetic, fuels, etc.

New carpet: latex is used for the carpet's backing with is a toxic chemical such as formaldehyde and acetaldehyde. The largest release of VOCs will occur in the first 72 hours after installation, but low levels of formaldehyde may continue to be emitted for years.

Air Fresheners: may increase indoor air pollution with long-term exposure. I will start coughing long before I realise there in vicinity.

House Air quality: Try to avoid air fresheners, scented candles, incense, eucalyptus oil, aromatherapy oils. It is important to air your house daily for 5 minutes to clear house chemicals.

Other sources of VOCs After decorating your house chemicals can often be floating in the air for a while as a result of the use of oil-based paints, here are a few of them-glues, floor varnishes, chipboard and treated. New furniture emits smell so if you can air the area for a few days all the better. Flatpack furniture: from China can cause very high formaldehyde emissions (VOC emissions), whereas IKEA is fine as they keep to European standards.

New and used cars are valeted with lots of chemicals, making them quite toxic to people with Salicylate intolerance. It's also advisable to avoid car washes, as they're full of chemicals and anti-freeze.

HOW TO REDUCE VOCs

Shops have a mirage of smells so if you notice strong smells such as perfume, then you should leave immediately, which should help you avoid getting unwell.

Have a well-ventilated area when using these chemicals and use according to manufacturer's directions.

Some environmental VOCs: gasoline, benzene, coal tar, oil, styrene (carpets), tetrachloroethylene (dry cleaning).

Benzene: this is a natural factor of crude oil and is found in tobacco smoke, stored fuels, paint supplies, thinners.

You can reduce levels of exposure to benzene by eliminating smoking within the house, ventilation during painting, discarding paint, fuels that will not be utilized directly.

Good house plants These will aid air-purifying the air of these chemicals. NASA researchers suggest that these plants are being an air-purifying champion: mother-in-law's tongue-(Sansevieria), spider plant (-Chlorophytum comosum), peace lily –(Spathiphyllum).

SOURCE: *Autoimmune disease -Xenobiotic exposures can induce autoimmune disorders, which sometimes have a genetic predisposition.
HTTPs://www.nap.edu/read/1591/chapter/6#60. Very little research has been done so that and we do not know the extent to which apparently spontaneous autoimmune disorders are influenced by environmental factors. If it is found that significant percentages of human autoimmune disorders are environmentally related and that these diseases can go into remission by removing the incriminated chemical or by reducing exposure to it.*

SENSITIVES TO CHEMICALS IN TEXTILES

Azo Dyes can cause a reaction for some salicylate intolerant

There have been increased reports of sensitivities to chemicals in textiles, leading to allergic dermatitis.

Clothes- Natural vs. Synthetic: textiles can be natural, synthetic or a mixture of both.

Synthetic fibre: is produced entirely from chemical substances include nylon, acrylic, polyester, polymers. Polyester does not stretch, absorb perspiration, or breathe which increases the danger of soaking up toxic chemicals.

Natural fibre: products are 100% obtained from either animal (wool and silk) or plants, cotton plant, linen (flax plant). Linen is known to be the world's strongest natural fibre, last a long time is thicker than cotton and has the natural ability to prevent bacterial growth.

Cotton fabrics can be very soft and better than other plant fibre. Yet it is worth mentioning that some people react to contact with wool.

Some chemical additives in clothes that cause reactions

Azo Dyes can cause a reaction for some salicylate intolerant. The dyes are found in the 100% acetate and 100% polyester, formaldehyde resin is used to finish fabric, tetrachloroethylene from dry-cleaned clothing can also produce problems.

Reaction to textile: This is rare, with immediate response to fabric fibres, with wheals, rash, respiratory and circulatory problems and rarely in severe cases some dyes can cause anaphylactic shock.

Reduce reactions: by washing new clothes before wearing them. Also, try avoiding polyester, acrylic, rayon, or nylon, and products labelled stain or water-resistant. Buy natural fibres, cotton, linen, silk.

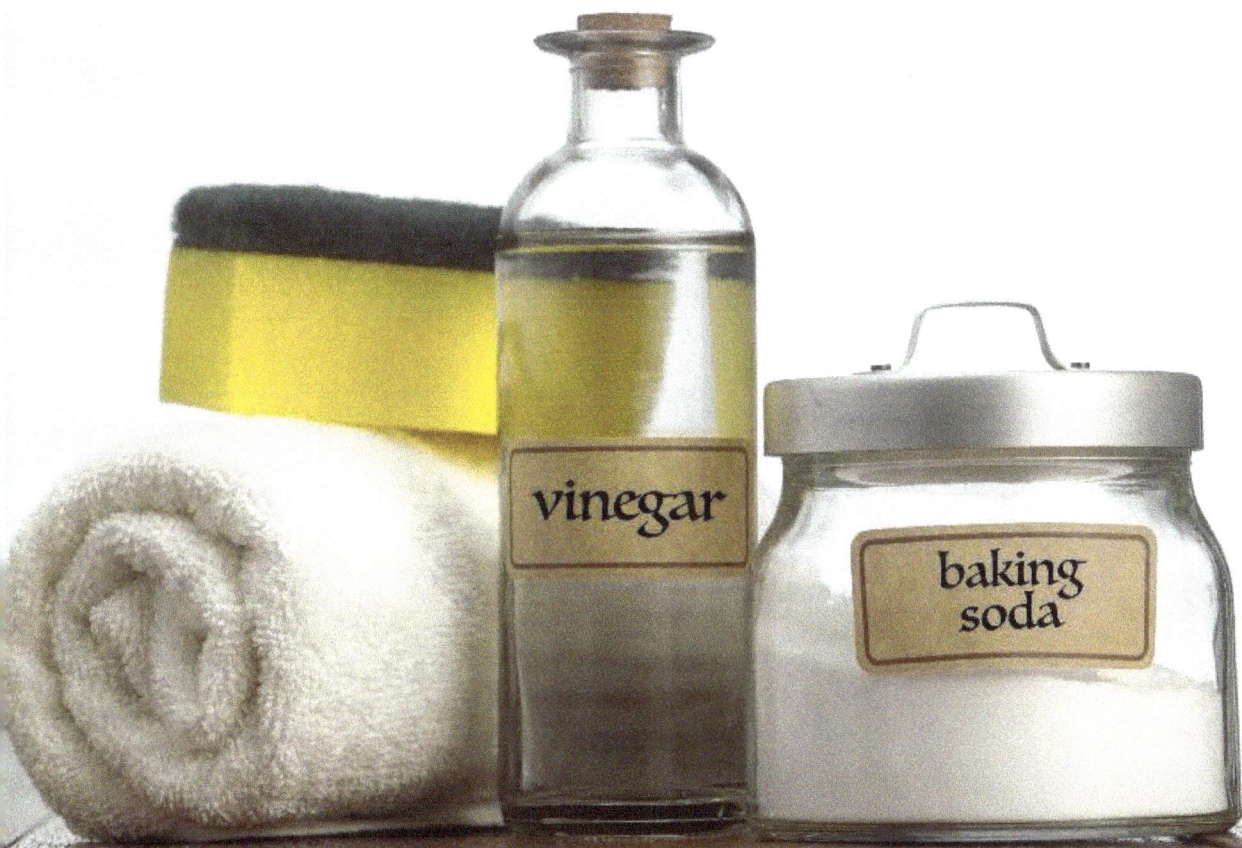

NATURAL & HOME MADE

PRODUCTS

HOME-MADE PRODUCTS

Man made products often have salicylates

Baking Soda Shampoo Baking soda is great for treating dandruff and absorbing excess oil. Method: Place the baking soda in the bottle, add 250 ml of previously boiled cooled water. Shake well. Gently massage into the hair and scalp and leave for a few minutes, rinse well.

Lime juice rinse Lime juice makes an excellent clarifying hair rinse. It helps rid your hair of any build-up and re-establishes the pH balance of your scalp. Method: mix 2 tablespoons lime juice and 250 ml water. To use: Pour the rinse over your hair and gently massage it into your scalp and leave for 5 minutes, wash off with plain water.

How to apply egg on hair Method: put an egg into a squeezable bottle and give it a good shake. In the shower wet your hair with *cool water, squeeze* the egg mixture all over your scalp. Leave on for 1-3 minutes, then wash well with cool water.

Rhassoul clay shampoo. Rhassoul clay is a mineral-rich mud and has been employed as a shampoo and hair wash since ancient times. It has saponins that make it soap-like when mixed with water. It is also natural conditioner, hair and body wash, face mask and natural Exfoliator. Safe for all skin types, even sensitive, dry skin or eczema, psoriasis. Method: use *non-metal utensils* when handling Rhassoul clay because the metal reacts with the minerals in the clay. Mix two tablespoons of clay with cold water into a paste, massage into wet hair and leave for 5 minutes then wash well.

Banana hair mask for dry & dull hair Bananas are an ideal base for a mask because they're charged with vitamins, minerals, antioxidants, and vitamin C and healthy oils that can moisturize and tone up your hair. Method: Mix and blend one ripe banana, 2 tablespoon sunflower oil, 2 tablespoon maple syrup, 1/2 cup yoghurt 1 teaspoon lime juice (optional). Apply this mask starting at the roots and working your way to the ends. Leave this on for about 30 minutes, then wash hair thoroughly and shampoo as usual then air dry.

Maple syrup for hair is beneficial to all types of hair with natural antioxidants. Method: apply 100 ml of maple syrup to wet hair. Thoroughly massage the scalp and put on a shower cap and leave in for 30 minutes. Rinse with tepid water and then shampoo as usual.

Homemade toothpaste Sodium Bicarbonate: this acts as an ideal mild abrasive and is alkaline, so it has the added benefit of helping to neutralize excess acid in the mouth. Apply about a ½ teaspoon of bicarb onto your brush and clean teeth, the paste will liquefy almost immediately when put into your mouth, so there is no need to add water.

Sea Salt: Sea salt has many minerals which strengthen gums, protect against tartar and bad breath, and possibly whiten teeth. It also works as a natural ant-bacterial agent and helps bring down swelling.

Bentonite clay: This is a fine powder and a mild abrasive, it is also alkaline, so it helps neutralize excess acid in the mouth, full of trace minerals.

Charcoal powder: brush with activated charcoal powder to kill bacteria, remove toxins and whiten teeth twice a week.

Shea Butter Moisturiser

Shea Butter-has the abilities to smooth away wrinkles and skin discolouration's. It can be applied straight from the package.

Soy Shea butter Moisturiser: use 10 oz. Shea butter, 6-ounce soybean oil, 2 tsp. Method: melt Shea butter over low heat, stirring constantly and whisk in soybean oil, and vitamin E drops. Whisk mixture until it is thick and creamy, and it forms soft peaks. Then put in storage jars.

Soy is rich in vitamin E, an antioxidant that moisturises your skin and provides protection against environmental irritants.

Vanilla Perfume Oil Vanilla extract: this has a potent vanilla scent when placed on your hotspot the wrists, neck and under your ears. Purchase a container to contain the perfume, or a sprayer bottle.

HOUSE CLEANING

Many of the chemicals used in the home have salicylates

List for cleaning Vinegar, bicarbonate of soda, limes, steamer, lye (soap), microfibre cleaning cloths. Air fresheners: use vanilla essence in water and spray.

Microfibre cleaning: these cloths lift off dirt, grease, and dust without the need for cleaning chemicals because they are formulated to penetrate.

Silver Microfibre clothes have the natural antibacterial properties of silver, to give the cloth the ability to self-purify. Glass/Windows: vinegar and water.

Polishes and metal cleaners

Brass cleaning: dust, then dip a soft cotton material into a variety of mild washing-up liquid and lukewarm water. With a slightly damp cloth gently wipe the brass surface.

Natural cleaner: dissolve a teaspoon of salt into a half cup of vinegar, add flour until the mixture becomes a paste. Rub gently into the brass, leave for about 10 minutes, then wash with warm water and buff dry.

Copper: soak a cotton rag in a batch of boiling water with 1 tablespoon salt and 1 cup white vinegar. Apply to copper while hot; let cool, then wipe clean.

Aluminium: clean with a solution of cream of tartar and water with a soft fabric.

Chrome: polish with vinegar.

Gold: clean with toothpaste, or a paste of salt, vinegar, and flour.

Silver: line a pan with aluminium foil and fill with water, add a teaspoon each of bicarbonate of soda and salt. Bring to a boil and immerse silver then polish with soft cloth.

Stainless steel: clean with a cloth dampened with undiluted white vinegar.

Cookware: mix 4 tbsp bicarbonate soda in 1 qt water, apply a soft cloth wipe dry.

Stainless steel sinks pour club soda on an absorbent cloth to clean, then wipe dry. To sterilise the sink, use boiling water.

Using Bicarbonate of Soda around the home It can clean without scratching. It is suited for use on aluminium, chrome, jewellery, plastic, porcelain, silver, stainless steel, and tin. It is an excellent deodorizer, and it can be utilised in the refrigerator, carpets, upholstery, drain. Also, use as a fabric softener by adding 2 cups of bicarbonate of soda to your clothes before starting the washing cycle.

CLEANING

Cookware: mix lime juice with sea salt and scrub also try baking soda and water made into a paste.

Oven Cleaning: make a paste of baking soda and water, apply the paste on the bottom of the oven and leave a few hours and clean.

Clean the Dishwasher: fill a dishwasher safe bowl or jar with 2 cups of vinegar and set on the top rack of the dish washer.

Lime Deposits in the kettle: reduce lime deposits by putting in 125 ml white vinegar and 2 cups water, and gently boiling for a few minutes. Rinse well with fresh water while the kettle is still warm.

Chopping block cleaner: rub a piece of lime across a chopping block to disinfect the surface. Use boiling water on the board to sterilise. Other- sprinkle baking soda on the surface of the cutting board, then work it into the surface stains with a lime or a gentle sponge. Apply coarse salt and scour the surface and leave for 5 minutes.

Toilet Cleaner: Use undiluted white vinegar, pour around the top of the toilet bowl, scrub.

Bicarbonate of soda- Put a cup into the toilet and let it soak for at least an hour. Pour in a cup of white vinegar, leave for 5 mins and flush. You can also dissolve steradent tablets in the lavatory to clean bowl because they have citric acid.

Bathroom: to remove lime scale, squeeze lime juice onto the affected areas, leave 5 minutes and then clean with a wet cloth.

Bath and Tile Cleaner: rub in baking soda with a damp sponge and rinse with fresh water.

For tougher jobs, wipe surfaces with vinegar first and follow with bicarbonate of soda as a scouring powder. (use sparingly as can break down tile grout)

Shower heads cleaning: fill a plastic bag with white vinegar and then tie the bag around the shower head and leave on for up to 12 hours and rinse.

Drain Cleaner: mix 1/2 cup salt in 4 litres hot water and pour down the drainpipe. For stronger cleaning, pour 1/2 cup bicarbonate of soda down the drain, then 1/2 cup vinegar, after 15 minutes, pour in boiling water to clear residue.

Mould and Mildew: Use white vinegar or lime juice full strength. Apply with a sponge. Cleanse from the Top Down: leave the floor or carpet for last.

Clean window blinds and shelves first and then work downwards. Allow time for the dust to settle before vacuuming. Rust Remover: Sprinkle a little salt on the rust, squeeze a lime over the salt, leave for 2 - 3 hours.

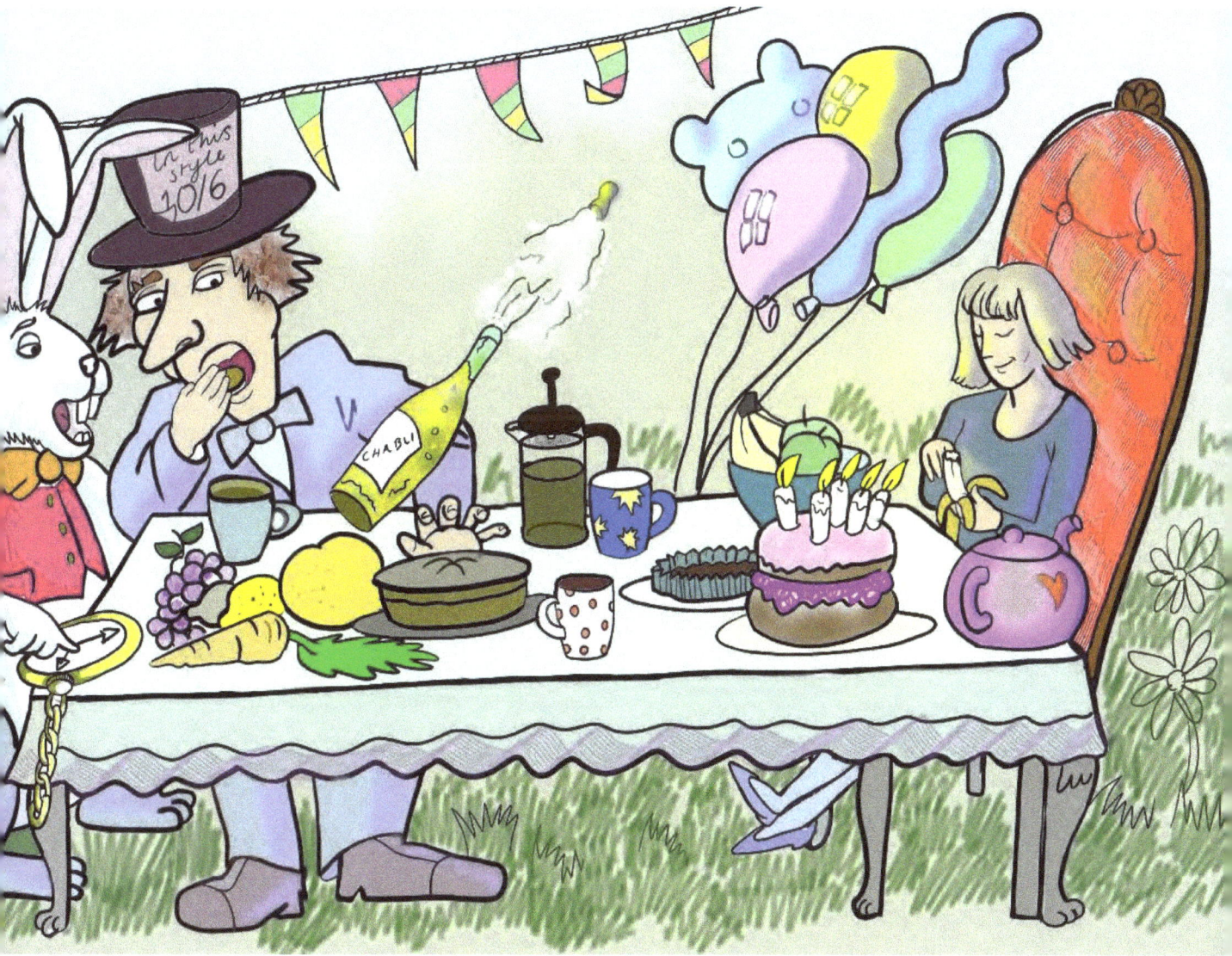

COOKBOOK

At the time of publishing all recipes are low salicylates but this may change with new research.

ROASTED BRUSSELS SPROUTS

500g brussels sprouts

3 cloves garlic, chopped

125g parmesan cheese, grated

3 tbsp sunflower oil or butter

salt

Method *Bake 200C/20-25 minutes*

Place the Brussels sprouts, cut in halves an oven-safe dish. Add the garlic, parmesan cheese, salt, followed by the oil. Toss to coat. Roast in the oven uncovered until crisp, brown and caramelized on the outside and tender on the inside. Serve with more grated cheese.

BRUSSELS SPROUTS PUREE

700g brussels sprouts

50g butter

1 tbsp maple syrup

1 tbsp lime juice

sea salt

Method

Cook brussels sprouts in boiling salted water until cooked. Put in blender and purée them with butter, salt, maple syrup and lime juice. Serve

ROASTED CABBAGE & BACON

1 savoy cabbage,

sunflower oil

4 slices thick bacon (has nitrites)

Sea salt

Method Bake 200/ Roast for 30 minutes

Cut the cabbage so you have eight wedges and place on a large roasting pan and drizzle lightly with oil and salt. Cut each slice of bacon into small strips and lay on top of the cabbage. Bake turning once.

Serve immediately; the wedges cool down fast.

ICEBERG LETTUCE & OYSTER SAUCE

500g iceberg lettuce

20 ml oyster sauce

1tsp dark soy sauce

1 tsp sugar

1tsp corn-starch

3 tbsp water

10 ml sunflower oil

4 cloves garlic, sliced

Method

Wash lettuce, then tears it into big pieces by hand. Bring a large pot of water to a boil. Turn off the heat and add the lettuce. Cover with a lid. After 1-minute, drain and place on a plate.

Mix oyster sauce, dark soy sauce, sugar, corn starch and water. In a pan, fry garlic in oil over a medium heat and turn off the heat when the garlic turns slightly brown. Add the mixture. Stir until well combined.

Pour the sauce onto the lettuce. Serve warm.

CREAMY LEEK GRATIN

2 tbsp unsalted butter

30g flour

500 ml whole milk

225g cheddar, grated

125g crushed bran flakes or

125g regular rolled oats

3 tbsp sunflower oil

6 leeks

salt

Method *Bake oven to 200/ 35 minutes.*

Sauce

Bring milk and butter to the boil, remove from heat add flour, salt and whisk, then bring to a boil. Remove from heat and stir in the Cheddar until melted.

In a small bowl, combine the bran flakes, oil, and salt.

Place the leeks in a single layer in the bottom baking dish. Cover with the milk mixture and sprinkle with the bran flakes mixture.

Cover the dish with foil and bake until the leeks are tender is bubbling.

ROASTED SWEDE

1 swede, peeled & cut into chunks

3 tbsp maple syrup

2 tbsp sunflower oil

Method *Bake 200 °C.* bake 45 mins

Heat the oil, add the swede and drizzle over 3 tablespoons maple syrup and toss well.

SWEDE LEEK & APPLE BAKE

25g butter

2 leeks, finely chopped

2 medium shallots

1 swede very finely sliced

2 apples, cored, halved & thinly sliced

75 ml water or homemade apple juice *See fresh apple juice recipe*

50g cheddar, grated

Method Bake *180 °C./cook 75 minutes*

Fry th*e* leeks, shallots in butter for 12 mins, add water, salt cook for 2 mins. Boil swede for 15 minutes, tray layer the swede, apple and leeks and shallots, finishing with swede. Cover with foil and bake for 45 mins. Remove foil, sprinkle with cheese, and bake for 15 mins until golden.

CREAM SWEDE

900g swede, small pieces

2 tsp sugar

30 ml cream

chopped fresh chives to garnish

sea salt

Method

Boil swede and sugar gently for about 40 minutes. Mash the swede, add salt cook until any excess moisture is gone, stir in the cream and garnish with chives.

ROASTED SWEDE & PARMESAN

1 large swede, cut into chips

1 tbsp sunflower oil

50g parmesan, grated

knob of butter

2 garlic

Method *Bake 220C bake 35 mins*

Put swede, sunflower oil, parmesan in tin., arranging in one layer. Sprinkle top with the remaining parmesan, dot with butter, then add the garlic cloves. way through cooking, until crisp and golden.

DAUPHINOISE POTATOES

1 kg of potatoes

3-4 garlic

300 ml double cream

300 ml milk

salt

50g gruyere grated

Method *Bake 160C/320F/1-1½ hours*

Thinly slice potatoes place in a bowl and rinse well to remove starch.

In a buttered oven proof dish put each layer of potatoes with crushed garlic and salt. Finally, pour over mixed milk and cream and put knobs of butter on top and slowly cook.

MUSHY PEAS

1 tsp butter

shallot diced

250g frozen or fresh peas

150 ml water, salt

Method

Fry shallots in butter. Cover the peas with water in a shallow pan and boil, then simmer for 3 minutes. Drain the peas add shallots and puree in a blender.

POTATO ROSTI CAKES

400g potatoes peeled and grated

1 medium egg, beaten

1 tsp plain flour

¼ tsp baking powder

2 shallots finely chopped

3 tbsp sunflower oil, for frying

Method

Squeeze any excess water out of the grated potatoes, then mix in a bowl with the egg, flour, baking powder, shallots.

Heat 2 tbsp oil in a large frying pan and spoon the mixture in to make 4, flattening them down with the back of a spoon into disc shapes.

Cook for 5 mins each side until golden brown and crisp, then drain on kitchen paper.

IRISH POTATO CAKE

500g leftover mashed potatoes

75g flour

30 ml milk

1 tbsp chopped chives

30g butter

Method

Combine mashed potatoes, flour, milk, and chives in a bowl and knead until smooth. Divide into 4 balls and flatten each into a 3-inch patty. Melt butter in a large frying pan, add the patties and cook until golden brown, 4 to 5 minutes per side.

CHEESE SHALOTT QUICHE

15g butter

4 shallots diced

75g grated cheese

300 ml single cream

4 Eggs beat

pastry case (see basic-pastry recipe)

Method Bake:30min /190 C.

Fry shallots in butter and cook until caramelised. Beat together eggs and cream, stir in cheese. Spread shallots in the bottom of pastry case then pour egg mixture in case.

ROASTED SHALLOTS

16 shallots

2 tbsp sunflower oil

2 garlic chopped

chives /Salt

Method Bake: 180 for 24 mins

Keep root of shallots attached and peal the rest to it does not fall apart. Place in roasting tin with chives oil, and garlic, salt

BLACK EYED BEAN SALSA

2 medium shallots, finely chopped

200g black-eyed beans, rinsed and drained

1 tbsp chopped chives

half lime, juice only

Method

Mix all the ingredients and serve.

PEAR & BEAN SALAD

4 canned pear halves chopped

45g munge bean sprouts

4 shallots chopped

125g tin red kidney beans, *rinsed*

100g soya beans, or use frozen, *rinsed*

125g sliced, cooked green beans

1 tbsp poppy seeds

50g sunflower oil

1 tsp sugar

1 garlic clove, crushed

1 tsp citric acid

half tsp sea salt

60 ml water

Method

Combine the peas, bean sprouts, green beans, shallots, kidney beans, and soya beans.

Dressing-combine the oil, citric acid, sugar, salt, garlic, and water and pour over the vegetables. Chill the salad for an hour before serving. Sprinkle with the poppy seeds -serve.

GREEK BLACK-EYED PEAS SALAD

1 can black-eyed beans

1 lime, halved

2 shallots, very thinly sliced

Salt to taste

Method

Drain and rinse the black-eyed beans, paper towel. Set aside.

Squeeze juice from one lime halves into a medium bowl. Slice the remaining limes in half into wedges and set aside.

Add the shallots to the bowl and toss with lime juice. Let sit for 5 minutes.

Mix and serve with lemon wedges for squeezing.

FETA SALAD

200g feta

splash lime juice

1-2 garlic cloves, crushed

100g hazelnuts

120g Iceberg lettuce

3 tbsp sunflower oil

salt

Method

Mix feta, lime, and garlic and leave to marinate. Mix a salad bowl lettuce sunflower oil, and salt. Crumble in the marinated feta and scatter the pomegranate seeds and grounded hazelnuts over. Serve immediately.

PASTA SALAD

250g pasta

2 shallots chopped

1 tbsp Greek yogurt

2 tsp chives

2 stick celery finely chopped

Salt

Method

Cook pasta, drain and rice in cold water. Mix all ingredients together.

COLESLAW

1000g thinly sliced cabbage

2 shallots, chopped

2 celery sticks

4 tbsp mayonnaise (homemade see basic)

2 tsp rice vinegar

Method

Place the cabbage, celery, shallots in a large bowl. Add the dressing ingredients and gently mix so that all of the shredded cabbage is coated with the dressing.

MEDITERRANEAN ROAST

2 shallots

3 large potato diced into cubes

swede diced into cubes

1 clove garlic diced

1 tsp of chives

125 ml water

2 tbsp bran oil

1tsp miso

Method Bake 180/45mins. Put all ingredients into casserole dish with water and sprinkle with oil and bake.

POTATO SALAD

800g potato

3 shallots, finely chopped

3 tbsp mayonnaise (see basic)

3 tbsp sunflower oil

1 tbsp rice wine vinegar

3 tbsp chives

1 boiled egg sliced (optional)

Method

Boil the potatoes in salted water for 20 mins, drain, then cool. Cut the potatoes into chunks and mix in shallots. Add enough mayonnaise to bind, then mix the sunflower oil and rice vinegar. Stir in the finely egg and chives and serve.

QUINOA SALAD

4 cups cooked quinoa

250g iceberg lettuce

250g cooked soya beans

125g diced shallots

1 large golden delicious apple,1/2-inch

6 tbsp sunflower oil

1 large lime, sea salt

Method

In a large bowl combine quinoa, lettuce, soya beans, shallots. Drizzle with oil, add lime juice and combine well, add salt Cover and chill for at least an hour. Stir and serve.

PEAR & CELERY SALAD

4 stalks celery

2 tbsp rice vinegar

30 ml maple syrup

2 ripe pears, diced

250g finely diced cheddar cheese

125g chopped pecans, toasted

6 large iceberg lettuce

salt

Method Blend vinegar, maple syrup and salt in a large bowl. Stir in pears; gently stir to coat. Add the celery, cheese, and pecans. Divide the lettuce leaves among 6 plates and top with a portion of salad.

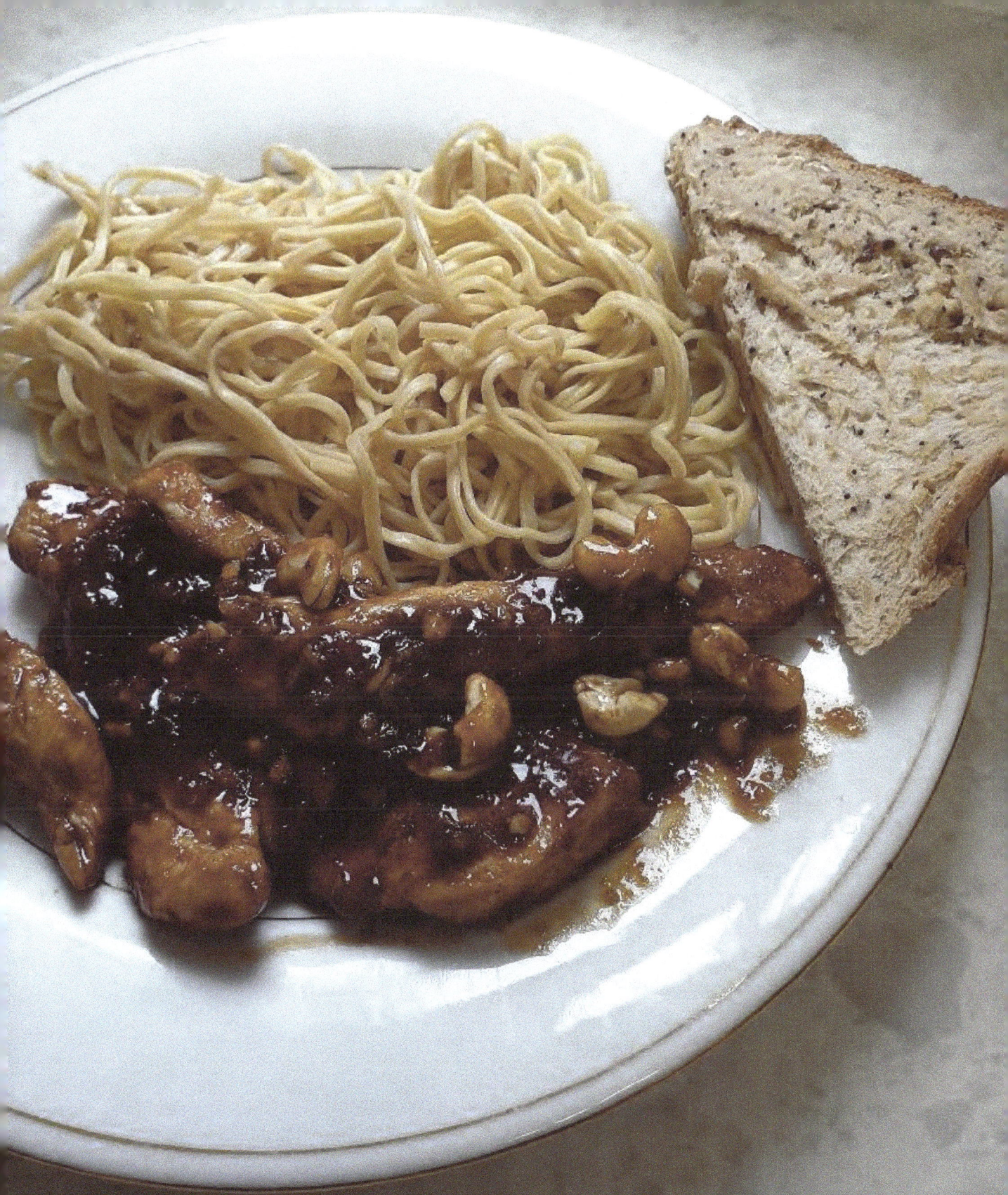

PASTA DISHES

CREAMY FRIED SALMON

225g egg tagliolini spaghetti

pinch of salt

4 boneless salmon fillets

200 ml cream Fraiche

4 tbsp chives

4 tbsp vodka

Method

Boil pasta with salt. Fry salmon for 3 mins each side. Remove salmon from pan add cream Fraiche, chives. Drain pasta, toss into the creamy sauce along with the pasta.

Serve- salmon and garnish with chives.

QUICK SALMON LIME SHELLS

415g can boneless skinless red salmon

250g yoghurt

400g dried shell pasta

1 lime juice (to taste)

1 tbsp chopped fresh chives

1 garlic clove, crushed

Method

Mix lime, chives, garlic, yoghurt and coat salmon with sauce and leave for up to 1hour.

Cook pasta and toss pasta shells and salmon pieces in the sauce. Serve with iceberg lettuce, celery. You can replace salmon with tin or fresh tuna.

SALMON & PASTA SHELLS

400g dried shell pasta

4x 150gr skinless fillet salmon

1 tbsp chopped fresh chives

30 ml sunflower oil

500 ml cream

4 shallots, thinly sliced

2 garlic cloves, crushed

1 lime juice (to taste)

225g fresh breadcrumbs

180g grated cheddar cheese

Method

Preheat oven to 180°/ bake for 25 minutes

Cook pasta in a large saucepan of boiling, salted water - drain. Steam salmon for 10-15 mins cool then flake. Heat oil in a frying pan over medium heat add shallots and garlic, stirring for 1 minute.

Add lime juice, cream, and salmon and reduce heat to low for 3 minutes or until heated through then add chives. Add mixture to pasta and pour into prepared dish. Combine breadcrumbs, cheese and sprinkle on top and bake until golden brown.

TUNA AND LIME BAKE

350g pasta shells

200g green beans

200g frozen peas

2 shallots chopped

1 tsp chives

200g can tuna drained

1 lime

300g crème fraiche

25g parmesan

salt

Method

Boil pasta for 8 minutes. Add the bean, peas and cook for a further 3 minutes until both the pasta and beans are just tender.

In a bowl flake the tuna in large pieces, add shallots, lime, crème fraiche, and salt.

Drain the pasta and beans, return them to the pan and toss with the tuna mixture. Serve with grated cheese.

QUICK PASTA CARBONARA

500g tagliolini spaghetti

1 tbsp sunflower oil

225g bacon rindless cut into 2cm

25g finely grated parmesan cheese

white sauce recipe. (see basic)

chives to serve

Method

Cook macaroni then drain. Grill bacon and put into pasta with white sauce, chives, and chess.

PHILADELPHIA PASTA

500g pasta

Philadelphia or a tub of cream cheese

2 large shallots

splash of milk

Method

Cook pasta as normal

Chop up the shallot onion and fry for 2 minutes, add half a tub of cream cheese and stir slowly until melted, then add milk to make the sauce a bit thinner.

Add the pasta and mix well and serve

MACARONI CHEESE

500g spiral or other short pasta

2 garlic, finely chopped

250g mature cheddar, grated

50g parmesan

250 ml cream

500 ml milk

50g butter

50g flour

crisps x 2pkt

Method *Bake 200C/45 minutes*

Boil 500g spiral or short pasta for 2 mins then drain under cold water.

Sauce

Boil milk, cream, and butter together. Then add flour and beat continuously until creamy and thick. cook garlic in butter for 1 minute and add to the sauce and simmer for 5 minutes.

Take off the heat, then stir in 250g grated mature cheddar and 25g grated parmesan.

Pour over pasta in prepared baking dish. Crush crisps and pour over top and bake.

Optional Cook some bacon and chop into pieces and put into pasta to cook.

LASAGNE, POTATO & BEAN

500g fake tomato sauce

2 canned red kidney beans

250g ricotta cheese

250g instant lasagne sheets

500g cooked potato

300 ml white sauce (see basic for sauce)

200 gr mozzarella cheese

Method Preheat oven to 180°C.

Puree the cooked potato. Place half the tomato sauce on the base of a lasagne dish and top with a layer of the lasagne sheets.

Cover the lasagne sheets with the red kidney beans and half of the ricotta and top with another layer of the lasagne sheets.

Spread over the remaining tomato sauce and another layer of lasagne sheets. Cover the lasagne with the potato puree and top with the remaining ricotta.

Top with another layer of the lasagne sheets and pour over the white sauce and sprinkle evenly with the mozzarella cheese.

Bake in a moderate oven for 45 minutes or until lasagne sheets are soft and topping is lightly browned.

POTATOES CABBAGE & PASTA

250g white potatoes/cooked

225g cooked pastas

clove garlic, minced

2 tbsp sunflower oil

1 tbsp butter

1 savoy cabbage, cored and shredded

125g grated cheddar cheese

Salt

Method

In a large pan fry garlic for 3 minutes, add the cabbage, salt, cook for 3 minutes, or until cabbage is softened.

Transfer the potatoes and pasta to the pan of cabbage along with the 1/2 cup of the pasta cooking water. Mix in the butter and cheese serve immediately.

SPAGHETTI & MEATBALLS

Use meatloaf recipe

tomato Sauce

fake tomato sauce 500 gr (see basic)

500 ml of water

400g dried spaghetti, salt

Method

Using wet hands roll into 20 balls, fry the meatballs on all sides until nicely browned.

Heat fake tomato sauce and water, add the meatballs and simmer for 10 minutes. Cook spaghetti until al dent.

Drain and serve the spaghetti topped with the meatballs and parmesan.

PEA BACON & RICOTTA PASTA

500g fusilli pasta

150g peas

1 tbsp sunflower oil

3 slices bacon, finely chopped (nitrates)

2 medium shallots finely chopped

500g ricotta cheese

2 tbsp chives

Extra parmesan to serve

Method

Cook the pasta according to packet instructions, add the peas about 1 minute before the end.

In a large frying pan cook bacon until browned then add shallots cook 5 minutes until tender. Reduce the heat to low, add Ricotta and cook for 1 minute.

When cooked, drain the pasta and peas, reserving 125ml of the cooking water. Add the cooked pasta and peas into the frying pan, along with the reserved cooking water, chives and Parmesan.

Serve immediately topped with Parmesan.

CHINESE STYLE BOLOGNESE

250g dried spaghetti

1tbsp sunflower oil

450g minced beef

4 shallots, finely diced

2 cloves garlic, minced

3 tbsp oyster sauce

2 tbsp soy sauce

1 tbsp sugar(optional)

25g frozen peas

450 ml water

2 tbsp arrowroot, mixed with 2 tbsp water

Method

Brown meat add the cooked shallots, garlic, and cook for 2 minutes then add boiling water. Bring back to boil and simmer. Mix in the oyster and soy sauces. Cover and simmer for 10 minutes then add the peas. Stir up the corn starch until sauce thickens.

Serve on Spaghetti.

SPAGHETTI BOLOGNSE

1 kg beef mince

400g spaghetti.

4 medium shallots finely diced

3 sticks celery, finely diced

4 garlic cloves, finely chopped

500 ml whole milk

15 ml of soy sauce

1tsp sea salt

1 tbsp butter

corn starch 15g to thicken sauce

To serve: 75g grated parmesan

Method s*erves 12 Cook for 1 hr 15 mins*

Melt butter adds shallots, celery sticks, garlic cloves and chives, fry for 10 mins. Add beef mince, salt and cook stirring for 4 mins until the meat is browned all over. Add milk, sugar, soy sauce and reduce to simmer and cover. Add rashers as required at the end and grated parmesan.

Spaghetti

Cook 400g spaghetti following the pack instructions. Serve with more grated parmesan, crusty bread.

EASY LASAGNE

1 tbsp sunflower oil

2 shallots, diced

2 celery diced

2 garlic cloves, finely sliced

500gr beef mince

500g fake tomato

400 water

1 tbsp maple syrup

500g pack lasagne sheets

50g Parmesan, grated

150g pack mozzarella, shredded

Method Preheat the oven to 200°C.

Fry shallots, and celery for 5 mins. Add the garlic and cook for 1 min, then add mince, and cook for about 6 mins until browned. Stir in the fake tomato purée and cook for 1 min.

Add 400 water bring to boil add maple syrup reduce to simmer for 20 mins. Layer up the lasagne in a baking dish, starting with a third each of the ragu, then the pasta, then the white sauce.

Repeat twice. Top with the Parmesan and mozzarella then bake in the oven for 40-45 mins, until piping hot and crisp.

Freezer: for up to 1-3 months.

FAKE MOUSSAKA

30g butter

4 shallots, chopped

1 tablespoon chopped chives

900g beef mince or lamb

50l (2fl oz) milk

1tsp salt

5 large potatoes, peeled and thinly sliced

Swede 600g thinly sliced, partially boil (15 minutes).

2 large clove garlic

1 tsp sugar

100g feta, crumble

fake tomato sauce 200 ml

Method

Use recipes -See white sauce recipe and Fake tomato sauce. Fry shallots in butter add garlic cook 2 mins, add lamb, and cook until brown.

Drain excess fat, add milk and fake tomato purée and cook for 1 min, add boiling water if necessary, simmer for 15 mins.

Arrange a third of the swede on the bottom of the baking dish. Top with half the mince mixture, then top with another layer of swede, followed by the final layer of lamb. Finish with a layer of swede or potatoes.

Sauce Pour the sauce over the top of the swede and sprinkle the surface with the remaining feta.

Cover with foil and bake in the oven for 35-45 mins then remove the foil and cook for a further 25-30 mins or until the top is golden.

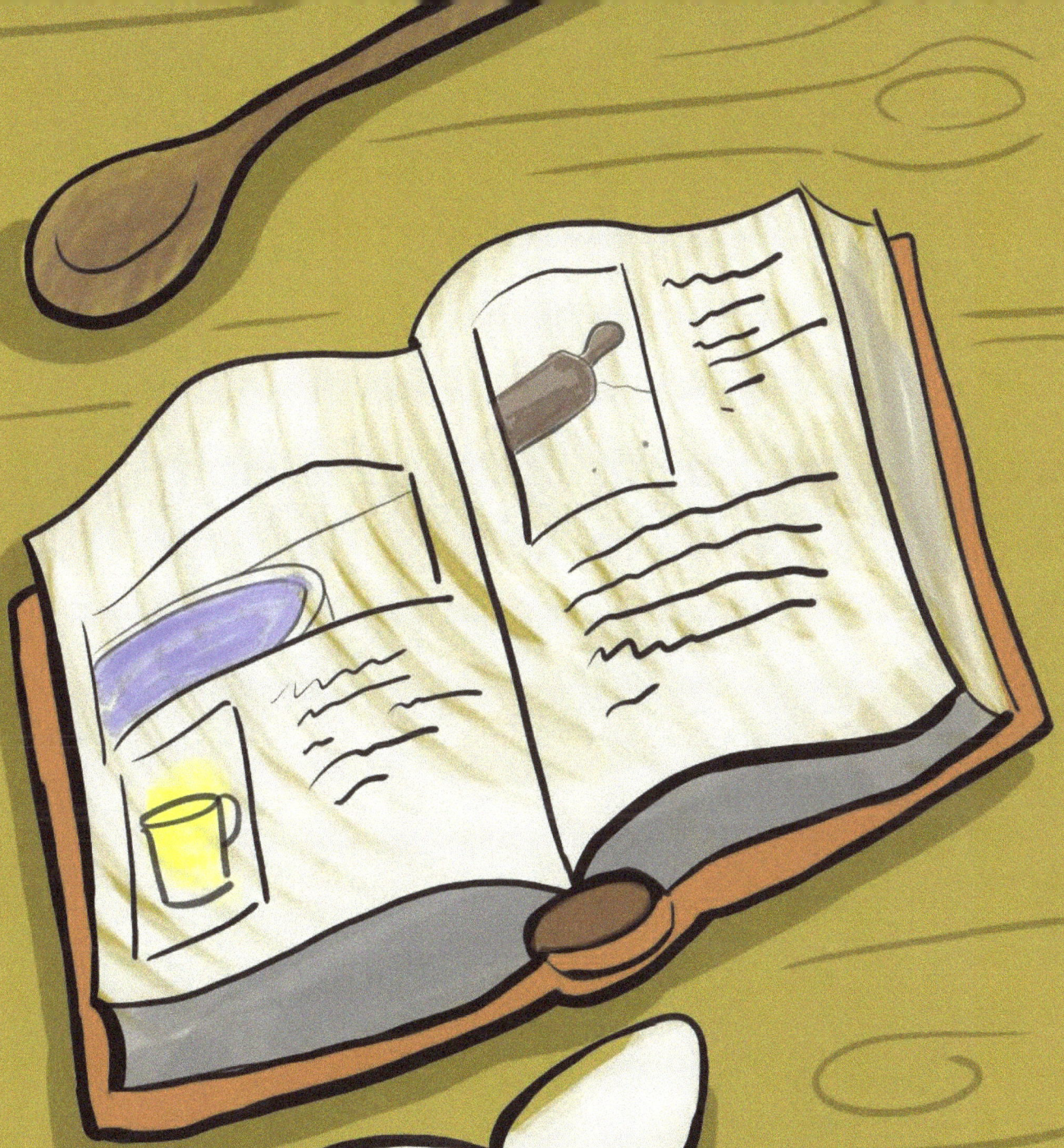

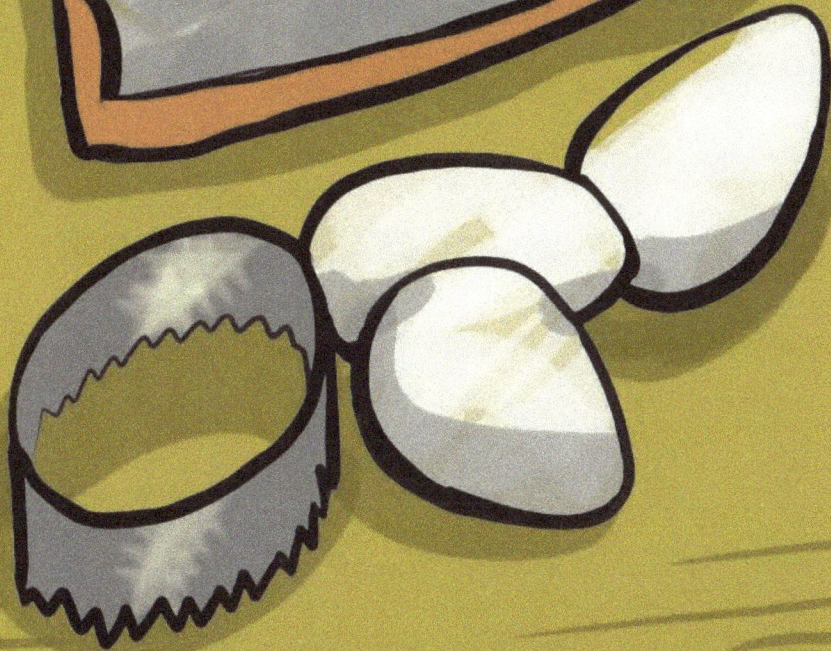

BREAD & PIZZA

SHALLOT GRUYERE PIZZA HAM

Pizza dough

4 shallots, sliced thin

1 tbsp of sunflower oil

225g gruyere cheese, shredded

8 thin slices ham or cooked bacon

1 small tub creme fraiche

Method *Bake 200, 8 minutes*

dough from bread chapter

Cook shallots in oil until they start to caramelize. Gently heat the creme fraiche until it is the consistency of heavy cream and then set aside.

Spread cheese on the crust to a half-inch from the edge. Layer the caramelized onions on top of the cheese, add the ham on top of the onions.

Generously drizzle the creme fraiche on top of the pizza. Bake or Grill on very low heat with the grill cover closed for just a few minutes being sure to char the bottom but not burn it.

CASHEW PIZZA

450g pizza dough

125 roasted cashews

2 small garlic cloves

125g sunflower oil

125g freshly grated Parmesan cheese

250g shredded mozzarella

150 Gruyère

salt

Method *Bake 200C 10 minutes*

In a food processor, pulse the cashew and garlic until minced and slowly add the oil until incorporated. Add the Parmesan cheese and pulse to combine with salt. Prepare dough base and brush with oil. Spread sauce and then top with chess and bake.

SCALLOP & BACON PIZZA

3 garlic cloves, crushed

125g sunflower oil

75g self-raising flour

375g whole milk

75g grated cheese

salt

450g pizza dough (see bread chapter)

4 slices thick-cut bacon (amines)

4 sea scallops 140g, sliced crosswise 1/4 inch thick

Method *Bake 200C*

Sauce: Cook the garlic in oil for about 3 minutes and then use white sauce recipe and whisk in the cheese and 15mls lime, and salt at the end. Transfer the sauce to a small bowl. Discard the garlic.

Dough: Roll out the dough into a 12-inch round. Transfer to the prepared sheet. Brush the remaining 15mls of oil all over the dough and spread the sauce evenly on top. Bake on the bottom rack of the oven for about 18 minutes, until the dough is almost cooked through.

Meat: Cook the bacon until golden and crisp and chop the bacon.

Topping: Top the pizza with the scallops and drizzle with olive oil. Bake for about 3 minutes, until the sauce is golden, and bubbling and the scallops are just opaque. Serve- bacon

THAI CHICKEN PIZZA

pizza dough

125g cashew sauce (*see sauces chapter*)

1 large chicken breast, chopped

15 ml sunflower oil

500g mozzarella

4 shallots

125g white bean sprouts

80g swede

30g cashews chopped

Method *Bake 200C/10 minutes*

Cook the chicken for about 5 minutes then coat with cashew sauce. Put in fridge. Spread 80g cashew sauce evenly over the prepared dough. Cover with 175g mozzarella.

Distribute half of the following ingredients over the top of each pizza, chicken, shallots, bean sprouts, and swede, add mozzarella. Bake or about 12 minutes until crust is golden and cheese is bubbly. Top pizza with cashew.

IRISH SODA BREAD

250g plain flour

250g wholemeal flour

100g porridge

1 tsp sodium bicarbonate

1 tsp salt

25g butter

500 ml buttermilk (or soured milk)

Method Bake oven 200 -30 mins

Mix dry ingredients then rub in the butter. Pour in milk mix with a knife. Shape with a cross on top and bake.

CHEESY SODA BREAD

500g self-raising flour

1 tsp cream of tartar

pinch of salt

175 ml milk

20 ml milk

20 ml sunflower oil

250g grated cheese

Method Bake oven 230 15 mins then reduce 200 for another 10/15.

Mix flour & cream of tartar and dissolve bicarbonate in milk, combine milk with dry ingredients. Add cheese knead lightly and divide it into balls roll and bake.

HOME MADE TORTILLAS

500gr plain flour

1/2 teaspoon salt

200 ml of water

3 tbsp oil or butter

Method

Combine flour and salt and stir in water and oil. Turn onto a floured surface, knead 10-12 times, adding a little flour or water if needed to achieve a smooth dough. Let rest for 10 minutes.

Divide dough into eight portions and on a lightly floured surface, roll each portion into a 7-ins circle.

In a large, oiled frying pan, cook tortillas over medium heat for 1 minute on each side or until lightly browned. Keep warm.

SIMPLE DOUGH FOR PIZZA

375g plain flour

1 tbsp caster sugar

7g dried active baking yeast

2 tbsp sunflower oil

225 ml warm water (45 C)

1 tsp salt

Method Cook:25min

Combine flour, salt, sugar, and yeast in a large bowl. Mix in oil and warm water. Spread out on a large pizza pan. Top as desired.

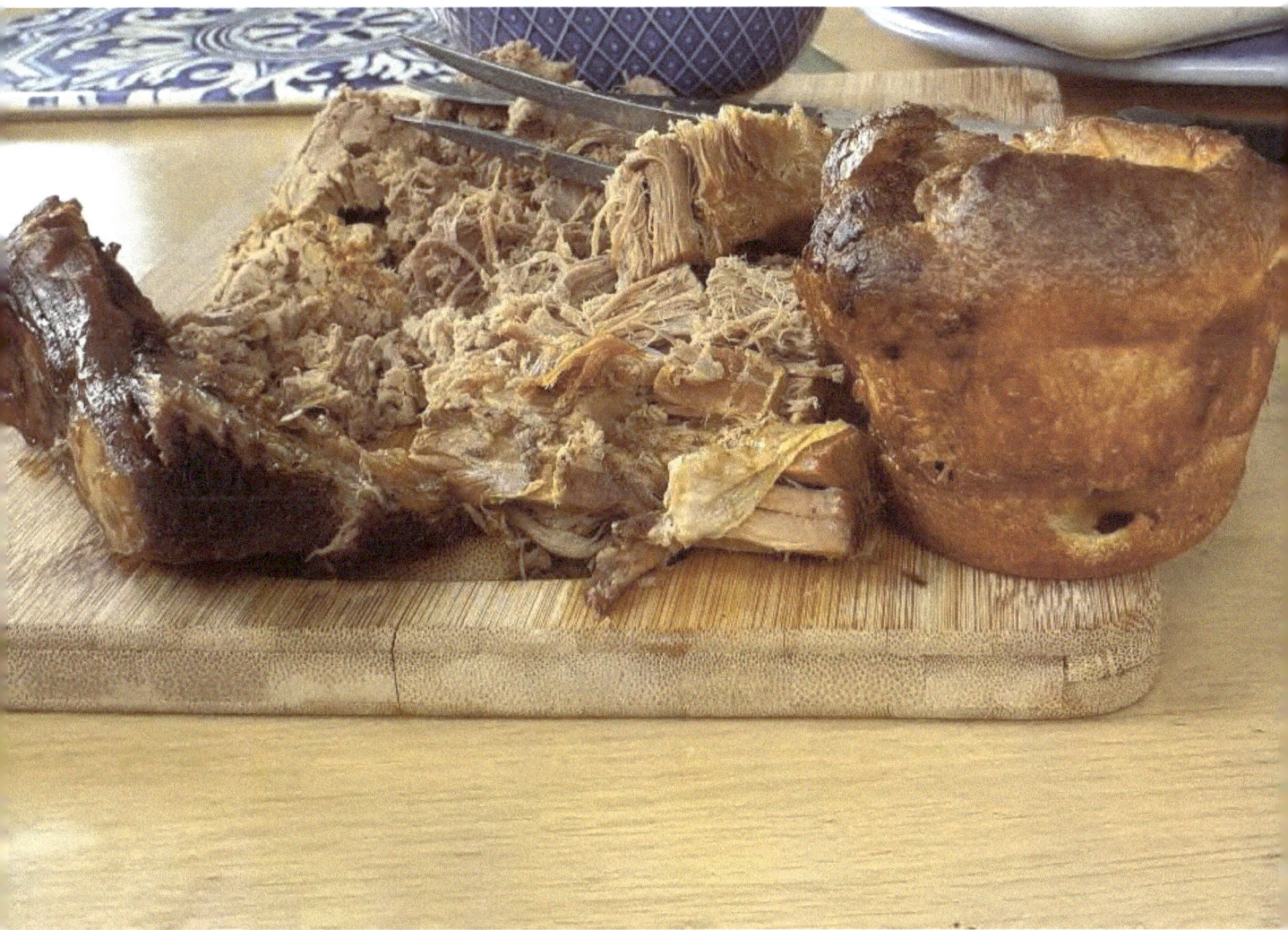

MAIN MEALS

LUXURIOUS FISH

400g fish pie mix (cod, salmon, etc)

200g frozen petit pois

200g grated cheddar

cook and mash potatoes

small bunch chives, finely chopped

Method *bake 20-25mins 200C*

Prepare white sauce (see white sauce recipe). Take off the heat and stir in the cheese, fish, chives, and peas.

Fry salmon and cod in butter and salt until they colour, pour into a dish and add white sauce. Put in baking dish top with the potato and sprinkle with cheddar cheese.

GARLIC BUTTER SALMON

680g salmon or trout

2 tbsp lime juice

2 cloves garlic, minced

3 tbsp melted butter

1/2 teaspoon salt

1 tsp chopped chives, for garnishing

Method

Melt the butter, add salt, garlic and squeeze the lime juice pour over the salmon. Fold the sides of the foil over the salmon and bake it.

SALMON PATTIES

1 can salmon, drained

2 shallots sliced

1 tbsp. chives

125g Panko breadcrumbs

1 tbsp lime juice

1 large egg, beaten

2 tbsp sunflower oil

salt

Method

To a large bowl, add first 8 ingredients. Form into 5, evenly sized patties. Place in pan heat oil.

Cook patties in batches until golden and crispy, 3-4 minutes per side. Drain on paper towels.

CHINESE FRIED FISH

250g cod

1 tbsp flour

2 tbsp sunflower oil

4 cloves garlic minced

2 scallions, sliced diagonally

Sauce

125 ml water

1 tbsp light soy sauce

2 tsp sugar

Method

Sprinkle fish with salt and flour to prevent, mix sauce ingredients in a bowl. S

tir fry garlic, and scallion, about 2 minutes. Add the fish and fry for 5 minutes each side. Place the fish on a serving plate.

Reduce the heat to medium and pour the sauce to the pan. Return the garlic and scallion into the sauce. Cook for a minute. Pour the sauce onto the fish. Serve rice.

OVEN FISH & CHIPS

900g potatoes cut into wedges

50g sunflower oil

75g fresh white breadcrumbs (or bran flakes or rice krispies crushed)

700g skinless boneless haddock or codfish fillets

2 tbsp flour, seasoned with salt 1 egg white, beaten

Method *Bake 12/15min 220 C*

Fish: Dip haddock or cod fillets into the flour, shake well to remove excess, then into egg white, and finally into the crumb mixture until evenly coated.

Place on a baking sheet sprayed with cooking spray and cook until golden brown. Serve with chips.

Bake for 35 mins/ 200°C Chips: cut the peeled potatoes into thick chip wedges.

Place on the baking tray and drizzle with sunflower oil, season to taste, turning halfway through cooking.

CREAMY FRIED SALMON

225 egg tagliolini spaghetti

4 boneless salmon fillets

200 ml cream Fraiche

4 tbsp chives

4 tbsp vodka

pinch of salt

Method

Fry salmon for 3mins each side add cream Fraiche, chives. Drain pasta, toss into the creamy sauce along with the pasta. Serve pasta top with salmon and garnish with chives.

MAPLE SYRUP SALMON

65g maple syrup

2 tbsp soy sauce

1 tbsp oyster sauce(optional)

1 crushed garlic

Method *bake 20mins/200 C*

Mix maple syrup, soy sauce, garlic together. Place salmon in the baking tray and coat with the maple syrup mixture.

Marinate salmon in the refrigerator 30 minutes.

Bake salmon uncovered 20 minutes, or until easily flaked with a fork.

GOUJONS O SOLE

50g plain flour

300g skinned lemon sole fillets (or any white fish), sliced into strips

1 large egg, beaten

50g breadcrumbs

Sunflower oil to drizzle

Sea salt

Method

Mix the flour and seasoning coat the fish strips in the seasoned flour, egg and then breadcrumbs. Arrange in a single layer on the baking sheet.

Drizzle the goujons with a little oil and bake for about 10 mins, turning over halfway

Salsa sauce: Use fake tomato sauce and add lime juice.

Serve the baked goujons immediately with the salsa.

TRADITIONAL IRISH STEW

950g diced fillet lamb

1.2 kg or 8 medium potatoes

6 large shallots

2 celery

1 tbsp snipped fresh chives (optional)

1-litre water to cover meat.

sea salt

Optional

1/2 of cabbage, thinly sliced

swede optional

Method *Cook 90 mins/ serves 6*

Immerse meat in pot and boil, skimming off all the impurities from the surface. Add sugar, salt, potatoes, shallots, celery on top of the meat. Bring to boil and simmer until cooked.

To thicken stew when it has cooked put 1 tablespoon of cornflour with a small amount of water mix then add a small amount of juice from stew then stir back into the stew and serve.

Tips for Stews: because you are using a lot of fresh ingredients there is no need for stock.

Thickeners: pearl barley, rice, beans and lentils, potatoes.

Rich texture: If you're browning meat or frying onions, coat it in seasoned flour first.

BEEF STROGANOFF

900g rump, sirloin or fillet beef trimmed and cut into 1cm strips

250 ml of water

1 tbsp chopped chives

80g flour

1 tbsp butter

Sauce: 250 ml crème Fraiche or cream

20 ml maple syrup

300g shallots

2 clove garlic crushed

30g butter

Method Sauce:

Fry the shallots in butter for about 10 mins, add garlic cook for 2 mins stir in the crème fraiche/cream and maple syrup and lime.

Meat: Dip and season beef in a bowl with 1 tbsp plain flour a big pinch of salt the, add the steak to pan, fry for 3-4 mins, then add the shallots back into the pan. Whisk crème fraîche, and water together, then stir into the pan. Cook over medium heat for about 10 mins.

Sprinkle with chives serve with rice, egg pasta, noodles, with some green vegetable. or sautéed potatoes.

MEATLOAF

800 gr beef mince or lamb

1 tbsp sunflower oil

1 large celery

1 tsp salt

2 egg

4 shallots, chopped

3 clove garlic

milk 60 ml as needed

250g dried breadcrumbs, or bran flakes

2 tsp soy sauce

Other: 250gr shredded Cheddar cheese, sugar 2 tsp

Method *Bake 180 C /1 hr* Optional: 1 golden delicious apple grated, 2 tbsp brown sugar

Mix milk with breadcrumbs then combines with all the other ingredients. Place in a lightly greased loaf tin and bake. Keep meatloaf in air-tight containers in the refrigerator for up to three days.

MINI MEATLOAVES

500g beef mince

175 ml milk

110g grated cheddar cheese

40g porridge oats

150 ml fake tomato ketchup

4 tbsp dark brown soft sugar

1 egg

salt

Method Bake 180C /45 minutes.

Using wet hands, combine ingredients thoroughly, shape into balls and place in a 12-muffin tray.

Serve with mashed potatoes, lettuce or other green vegetables.

Freezing tip: Freeze these mini meatloaves either before or after baking and freeze for up to one month.

CANTONES BEEF RICE

1 tbsp sunflower oil

450g beef

1 large shallot, finely diced

3 cloves garlic, minced

1 tbsp Shaoxing wine

500 ml water

3 tbsp oyster sauce

2 tbsp light soy sauce

1 tsp dark soy sauce

250g frozen peas

2 tbsp corn starch

Method

Heat the oil to a wok, add the beef and cook until slightly browned. Add shallot, cook until translucent, and then add the water. Bring to the boil then simmer. Stir in the oyster and soy sauces. Cover and simmer for 10 minutes, then add the peas, and stir-fry for one minute. Mix corn starch, with 2 tablespoons water, add to pan stirring constantly until thickened. Serve with rice.

HAMBURGERS

600g minced beef

4 shallots or leeks chopped

3 celery chopped (optional)

15g chopped chives

1 clove garlic

2 eggs beaten

25g rice krispies or bran flakes finely crushed

30g maple syrup (optional)

60 ml milk

sea salt

Method

Mix all the ingredients. Roll into 6 balls. then flatten into 5mm thick and cooks for 20mins.

Serve with home-made rolls, chips and Iceberg lettuce.

CHEESEBURGER

500g minced beef

2 tbsp sunflower oil

4 shallots chopped

2 eggs beaten

To Serve

4 soft hamburger buns

4 slices cheddar

fake tomato sauce

sea salt

Method

Combine mince, shallots, eggs salt and divide the minced into four equal portions and shape into patties. Chill in the fridge for at least 10 minutes.

Fry or grill. Add a slice of cheese to the cooked top of the patties until the cheese is melted.

Serve in a bun with fake tomato sauce.

PS: you can add flour if need to hold them together.

CABBAGE MINCE ROLLS

500 g minced meat

3 shallots finely chopped

80g raw rice

3 tbsp chopped chives

12 cabbage leaves

Method *Bake 190C-1 hr 20 mins*

Mix meat, rice, egg, shallot, salt. and spoon into the centre of each of the cabbage leaves and enfold meat. Place folded side down in a greased baking dish.

Sauce-Mix together brown sugar, lime juice, and fake tomato sauce. Pour over rolls, cover tightly, and bake for 1 hour then uncover and bake 20 minutes longer.

1 beaten egg

1 tsp salt

For sauce:

125g brown sugar,75g lime juice, 250g fake tomato sauce

COTTAGE PIE

600g beef mince

500 ml water

50g sunflower oil

2 shallots, finely chopped

2 garlic cloves, finely chopped

50g plain flour

30g soy sauce

frozen peas

1 tbsp flour

50g strong cheddar grated

Mashed potatoes

Method *Bake 180 C / 20 mins*

Cook and mash potatoes add grated cheese and set aside. Fry shallots add beef mince and brown.

Stir in flour and cook for 1 minute, add soy sauce, water, frozen peas, boil, then simmer for 5 minutes.

Place in casserole dish. Top with the cheesy mashed potato mixture and sprinkle grated cheddar cheese over the top.

LAMB MEATBALLS

400g lean lamb mince

400g tin of chickpeas

350g fake tomato sauce

20 medium saffron threads

5 ml sunflower oil

2 shallots

2 cloves of garlic

Salad: 125g celery, lettuces, 50g fake tomato sauce, 1 tbsp sunflower oil, 1 lime

Method

Meatballs: Mix the mince with salt, divide into 4, with wet hands roll each piece into 4 balls, fry in oil until dark golden.

Sauce: In a cup put the saffron and cover with boiling water and leave to soak. Fry shallots in oil, add garlic and fry for 40 seconds, add the saffron with its water, the drained chickpeas, fake tomato sauce cover and bring to the boil and pour over meatballs.

Salad: Roughly chop and mix all the salad vegetables for the salad, add oil, lime juice.

Tortillas: Microwave (800W) the tortillas for 45 seconds. Serve it all with lime wedges and a scattering of chives. Buy from the shop or make from recipe under bread chapter.

To serve: 60g natural yoghurt, 8 small whole wheat tortillas, 1 tbs lime juice

KOFTE LAMB

400g lean lamb mince

25g grounded hazelnuts

1 tbsp golden syrup

150g of couscous

sunflower oil

Salad:

150mls fake tomato sauce, 4 heaped tbsp yogurt, ½ an iceberg lettuce,

1 shallot, 1 celery, 2 lime, 40g feta cheese

To serve: 4 Pita breads

Method

Mix the mince with salt then with wet hands divide into 8, shape into sausages. Frying in oil until dark golden, drain excess fat from the lamb, add hazelnuts, chives, and golden syrup and turn the heat off. Make couscous.

Salad: Grate the shallots and celery, salt into a bowl, add fake tomatoes and lettuce. Mix the yoghurt in a bowl with lime, then drizzle over the lettuce and crumble over the feta.

Serve: Pop the pita in the microwave (800W) for 45 seconds to warm through, fluff up the couscous, serve with lime wedges.

LAMB & PAWPAW

700g of boneless leg of lamb

1 tsp of brown sugar

2 tbsp of sunflower oil

4 clove garlic

8 shallots

few slices of papaya

400 ml condensed milk

salt

Salad: 1 papaya,2 tbsp lime juice,1 tbsp soy sauce

Method

Cut the lamb into 3cm cubes and mix with papaya. Blend the garlic, shallots and fry a couple of minutes and then add the lamb, sugar, and salt to taste.

Bring to boil and simmer for 30 minutes. Add condensed milk, simmer until meat is tender.

Salad: Skin and chop papaya into 3cm (1¼in) slices. and mix with soy sauce, lime juice.

Serve: Garnish lamb with papaya salad and serve.

CHINESE PORK & RICE NOODLES

Pork Dishes

140g rice noodle

250g pork mince or thin strips

250g mung bean sprouts

2 tbsp maple syrup

1 tablespoon sugar

15g rice wine

15g dark soy sauce

15g light soy sauce

50 ml water

chives chopped

3 garlic cloves

Method m*arinate overnight*

Whisk all the sauce ingredients together soy sauce, water, oil, maple syrup, sugar, rice wine, garlic. Marinate the pork in the sauce overnight or for at least a few hours. Discard excess and cook pork until brown and then add mung bean sprouts Serve with noodles.

CORNISH PASTRIES

Cooked chicken lamb beef etc. Pastries from pastry recipe

Method *Bake at 180 C 30 mins*

Use pastry recipe. Divide the dough into 14 circle pieces. Filling for pasties. Use cooked chicken lamb beef etc.

Spoon the filling onto the middle and brush the edges with egg and fold over. Cut a small hole in the top and brush with egg then cook. Serve vegetables or salad.

Serve with pear sauce (see sauces). Can be frozen.

CHINESE STYLE PORK

550g pork tenderloin

30g sugar

30g maple syrup

25g light soy sauce

25g oyster sauce

1 tsp sunflower oil

1 clove garlic, crushed

2 shallots, diced

salt

Method *Bake 200/ 30 minutes.*

Combine all ingredients and marinate 2 hours. Serve with rice & peas.

PORK MASCARPONE

2 x 225g Pork Tenderloin

4 bacon

250g tub Mascarpone cheese

juice of one lime

chives

1tsp salt

Method *Bake 200°C 30mins*

Cut incisions along the pork from the top to the bottom, but not all the way through.

Mix the mascarpone, lime, salt, and chives. Fill the pockets with half of the mascarpone mixture, then wrap the pork with bacon, and place in roasting tin in oven.

Add the remaining mascarpone mixture into a pan and add pork. Stir until well combined and heated through.

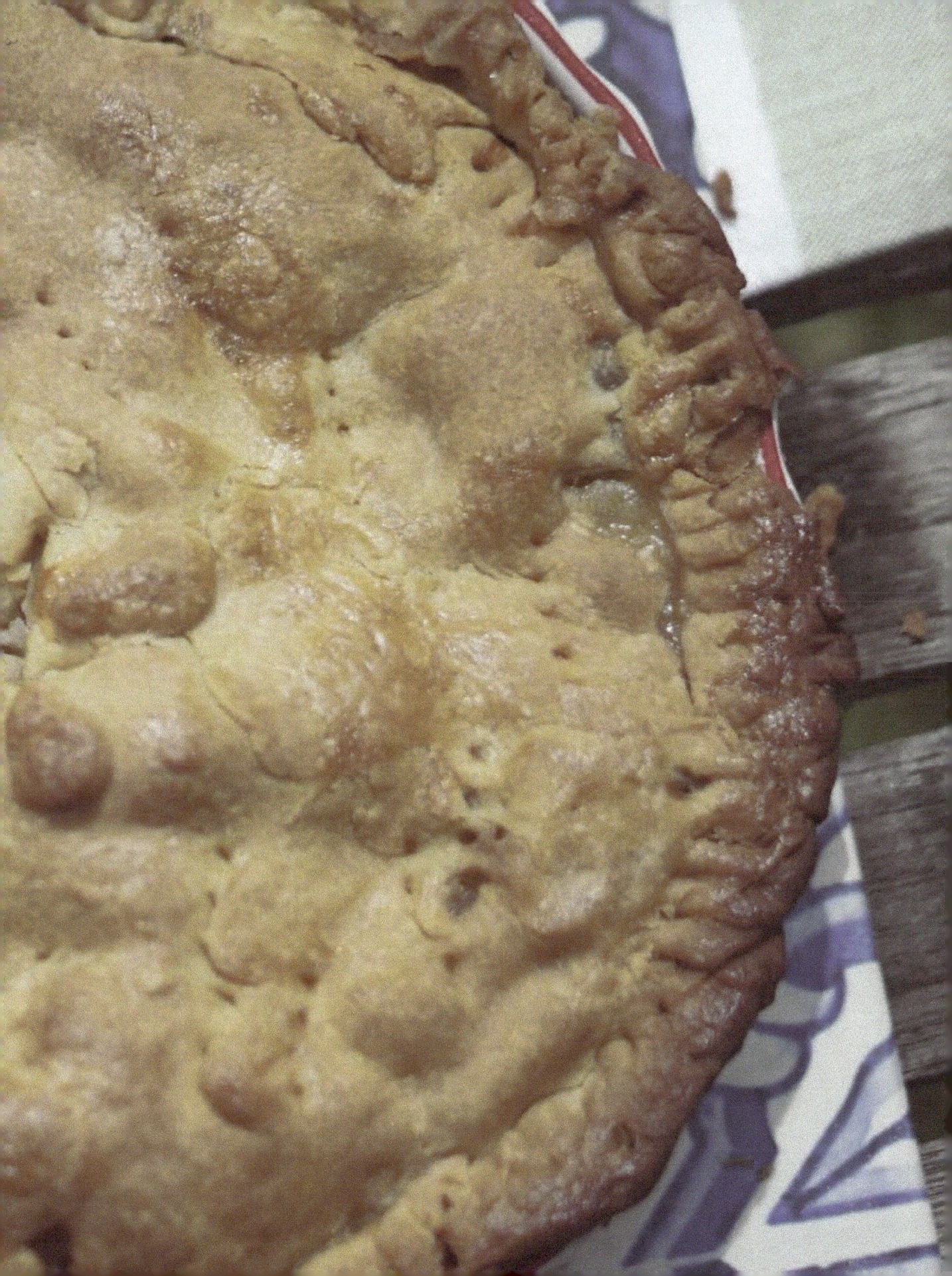

CHICKEN DISHES

CHICKEN MISO QUINOA

6 chicken fillets cut in small, long slices

shredded cabbage or 500g brussels sprouts

500g quinoa

Sauce:

1 tbsp white miso paste

2 shallots chopped finely

150g parmesan cheese

800 ml water

3 cloves fresh garlic (diced)

Method *Bake in the oven at 180C 1 hour. / serves 12*

Sauce: mix all ingredients.

Pour quinoa into a large casserole, lay chicken, and Brussels on top, then pour the sauce over this. Flip chicken breasts twice during cooking to prevent them from drying out.

CHICKEN IN BREADCRUMBS

125g fresh fine breadcrumbs (or rice krispies or bran flakes)

4 boneless and skinless chicken breasts, cut into strips

50g plain flour

3 eggs, beaten

2 tbsp sunflower oil

salt, to taste

Method Bake 190C.35 minute

Mix the breadcrumbs with salt. In another bowl place the flour another the egg. Dip the chicken pieces in plain flour, then in the beaten egg and finally coat in the breadcrumbs.

Shake off the excess and lay the chicken on an oiled baking tray. Drizzle the chicken all over with more of the oil and bake.

CHICKEN RICE BEAN BURRITOS

6 flour tortillas (see homemade recipe)

250g cooked rice

250g cooked chicken, shredded

250 shredded cheese blends

Refried beans

400g can black beans

(or red Kidney bean), drained & rinsed

2 tbsp butter

2 garlic

1/2 Lime juice

Method

Cook garlic in butter for 4 mins. Stir in beans and salt and cook for 5 mins. Squeeze in lime juice.

Preparation- Freeze: layer burrito starting with refried beans, followed by cooked rice, chicken, and cheese. Fold in the left and right sides of the tortilla and roll it up from the bottom, tucking the bottom edge under the filling.

Wrap in parchment paper and label. Freeze up to 1 month. To reheat from frozen, wrap the burrito in a damp paper towel and microwave for 2-3 minutes, flipping halfway or until the centre is hot. Let stand 1 minute before eating.

Salad: 4 tablespoons Greek yoghurt. Lime juice, chives, lettuce. Mix yoghurt, lime, chives.

Serve: Spoon into heated tortillas add lettuce grated cheese and add a spoon of yoghurt mix. Good for picnic

CHICKEN KIEV

8 chicken breast fillets

100g plain flour

225g breadcrumbs or bran flakes

75g parmesan, grated

4 tbsp sunflower for frying

4 egg, beaten

For the garlic butter:

4 garlic cloves, crushed

2 tsp finely chopped chives

200g butter softened

juice ½ lime (optional)

Method

Garlic butter: Place all the garlic butter ingredients in a bowl and shape into two sausages using cling film wrap and chill or freeze until firm. Can be made up to 3 days in advance. When firm, slice each into 8 even pieces. Set aside. Chicken: cut a slit into the side of each chicken breast to form a pocket then stuff garlic butter mix into chicken.

Breadcrumbs: Three bowls- first- mix the breadcrumbs and parmesan, second two-eggs, third mix the flour, salt. Dip each breast into beaten egg then in flour then in egg again, finally in the breadcrumbs.

Chill for at least 1 hr before cooking then places on a baking tray and cook. Freezing: Freeze each Kiev for up to 3 months and on the day that you make them. For best results, cook from frozen. Simply put them on a baking tray and cook as above, turning halfway through.

SIMPLE SOY CHICKEN

Chicken fillet x6

Sugar 60 g

Oyster sauce 60g

Soy sauce 120g

Method *Bake oven 180 / 30 mins*. Marinate for 2 hours or overnight. Remove from sauce place in tray and bake.

CHICKEN & BACON

4 chicken breast fillets

1 tsp chives

120g Philadelphia

4 bacon

Method

Cut a slit into the side of each chicken breast to form a pocket and spread the cheese into the middle. Wrap each chicken breast with 1 slice of bacon. Cook for 25-30 minutes. Serve immediately with potatoes and a green vegetable of your choice.

CRUNCHY CHICKEN

Crunchy Chicken

10 chicken fillets

250g bran flakes

50g poppy seeds

75g flour

75g water

2 eggs

salt

Optional- 65g cashews finely chopped

Method

Dust chicken with flour bowl then dip in egg bowl and finely water bowl.

Roll in combined bran, poppy seeds, nuts salt and refrigerate for 30mins. Spray chicken with oil and bake for 30 mins.

CHICKEN A LA KING

450g chicken fillets, thin strips

1 x celery thinly sliced

4 shallots finely sliced

1 tbsp sunflower oil

400 g rice cooked

White sauce:

125 ml fresh cream

350 ml milk

60g Plain Flour

60g Butter

Method

Cook the chicken strips add the shallots, celery and cook for another 5 mins.

White sauce

Mix cream milk butter in a pot bring to the boil, take off heat beat in flour return to heat and cook.

Mix chicken and sauce and bring back to boil. Serve - with rice.

CHICKEN QUINOA SALAD

6 chicken fillets cut in thin strips

30g lime juice

½ teaspoon sea salt

80g plain yoghurt

2 cloves garlic, minced

15g sunflower oil/bran oil

1 tsp maple syrup

rice vinegar

Iceberg lettuce

250g cooked quinoa

3 shallots

80g cashews

250g cubed fresh mozzarella

Method

Chicken- mix lime juice, sea salt pour over chicken set aside for 15 minutes then cook until golden brown and cooked.

Dressing: mix ingredients in bowl. In a large bowl combine lettuce, quinoa, shallots, and cashews. Divide mixture between four plates and top with chicken and mozzarella. Serve-drizzle with dressing and serve.

MAPLE CHICKEN ESCALOPE

500g chicken breast fillets, cut in horizontally slices

1 large pear, peeled, cored and quartered

75g maple syrup

1 garlic, finely chopped

1 tbsp salt

chives

Method *Bake 200C/ 1 hour*

Combine the maple syrup, garlic, salt and add the chicken and refrigerate overnight. Put chicken and marinade in a baking dish, place pear quarters around the chicken pieces.

Bake until chicken is cooked through, basting occasionally.

Serve: sprinkle with chives and serve immediately over rice.

CHICKEN PIE

6 slices fillet chicken

4 shallots or 1 leek, chopped

4 bacon cut into little pieces (nitrates)

60g Butter

Pastry (see pastry section)

Method *Bake 200C/25 minutes*

Use white sauce recipe see sauce chapter Cook chicken and then sauté leek, bacon when cooked add sauce.

Cover with pastry, making a vent in the pie top, and brush with milk. Bake until golden.

CHICKEN MASCARPONE SAUCE

6 large fillet chicken breasts

2 shallots chopped

30 ml bran oil

200g of fake tomato sauce (see recipe)

1 tsp salt

1 tsp sugar

250g mascarpone cheese

chives

Method

Fry shallots in oil for 5 minutes. Mix in the fake tomato sauce with the salt and sugar, bring to the boil and simmer for 10 minutes with the lid on, then 10 minutes with the lid off.

Take off the heat and blitz until smooth with a hand blender. Stir in the mascarpone, chives and set aside. Fry the chicken in oil until golden brown. Pour the sauce into an ovenproof dish then place the chicken breasts, on top and cook in the oven for 30 minutes

FAKE CURRY CHICKEN PAPAYA

6 chicken fillets

125g Flour

30 ml sunflower oil

2 pawpaw, ripe, medium

175 ml brown sugar

juice of 1 lime

1 tbsp arrowroot

30 ml soy sauce

salt

Method *Bake 80 C./45 mins* Place the chicken, salt, flour in a large plastic bag and shake until well coated. Shake off the excess.

Place in a large baking pan brush the top of the chicken with oil. Bake until golden on the outside.

Sauce: peel and seed the papaya, cut into cubes. Combine the juice, sugar, arrowroot, and soy sauce in a saucepan and bring to a simmer, stirring constantly, cook, until thick.

Remove from the heat and add the papaya. Spoon the sauce over the chicken and serve.

CHICKEN CASHEW

6 fillet chicken, cut into small slices

250g unsalted cashews

1 tbsp sunflower oil

30g cornflour

cooked rice or noodles

1 tbsp chopped garlic

150 ml of soy sauce

1 tbsp rice vinegar or rice wine

1 tbsp brown sugar

2 tbsp oyster sauce

2 tbsp maple syrup

pinch of salt

Method

Sauce: mix salt, sugar, garlic, oyster and soy sauce, maple syrup and rice wine. Allow marinating for 30 minutes. Season chicken with salt and cornflour in a bowl. Then cook with oil in the pan for 7 minutes or until brown then add cashews and sauce.

Serve with cooked rice or noodles.

LIME CHICKEN

4 skinless fillet chicken breasts

200 ml Greek yogurt

1 tbsp maple syrup

1/2 lime juice

1 small bunch chives chopped

Method *Bake 190°C /20 minutes*

Mix in the yoghurt, lime zest, maple syrup and pour over chicken. Marinate in the fridge for 2 hours or overnight.

Bake for about 20 minutes. Serve on rice or fried rice with chopped wedges, bean shoots, green beans, shallots, garlic, salt.

PASTA LIME CHICKEN

225 Tagliatelle pasta

15 ml sunflower oil

25g butter

4 shallots sliced

100g peas

1 clove garlic

100g lean ham diced (has nitrates)

225g chicken fillet cooked sliced

1 lime juice and salt

Method

Cook pasta. Then cook shallots, garlic in oil and butter for 4 mins and add peas stirring for another 3 mins.

Mix ham, chicken into the vegetable mixture along with pasta and lime. Return to heat cook for 4 mins, then serve.

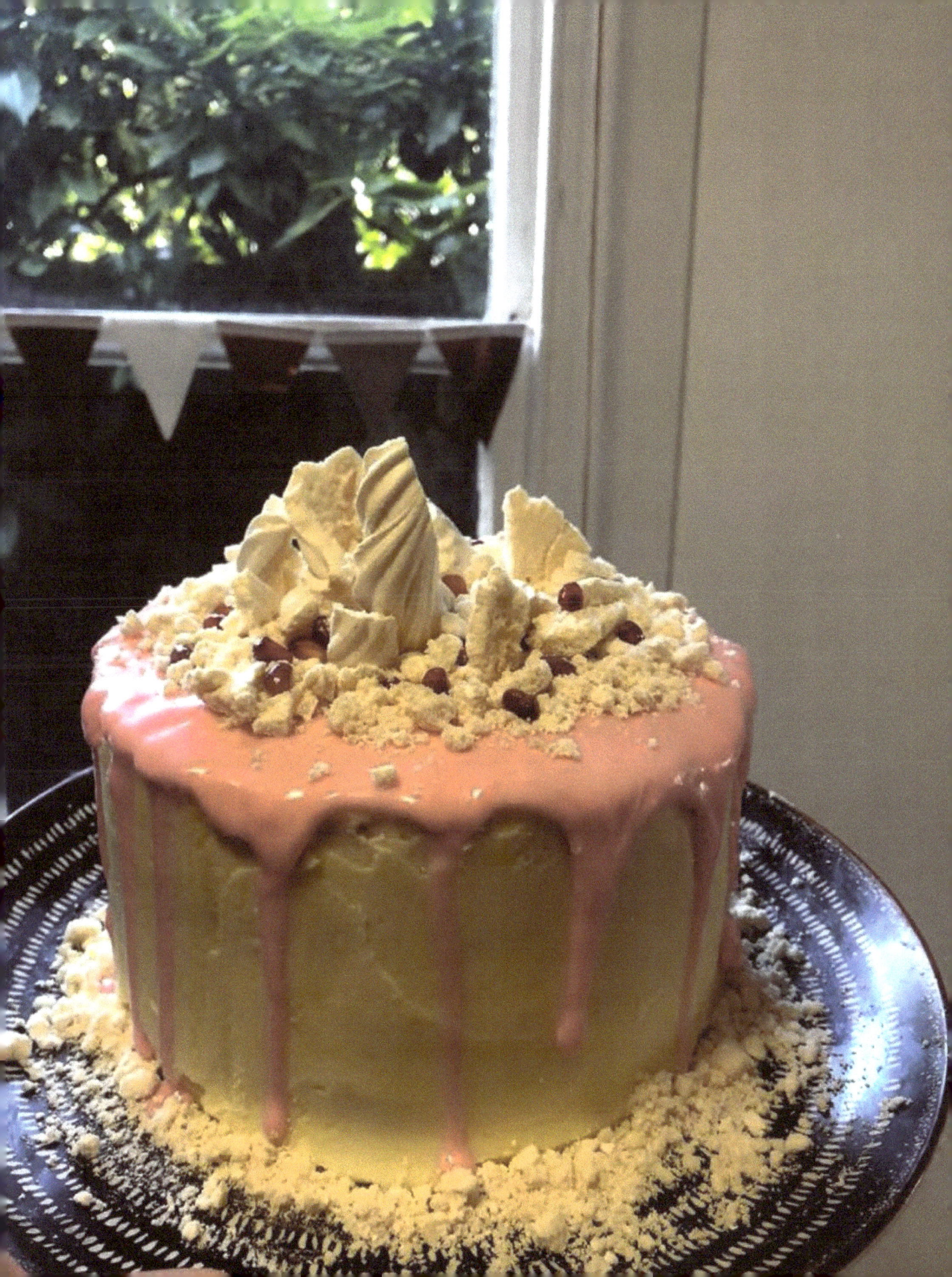

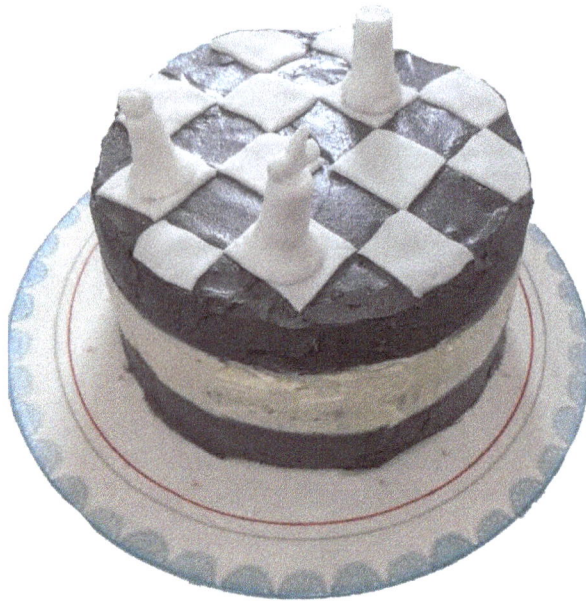

DESSERT DISHES

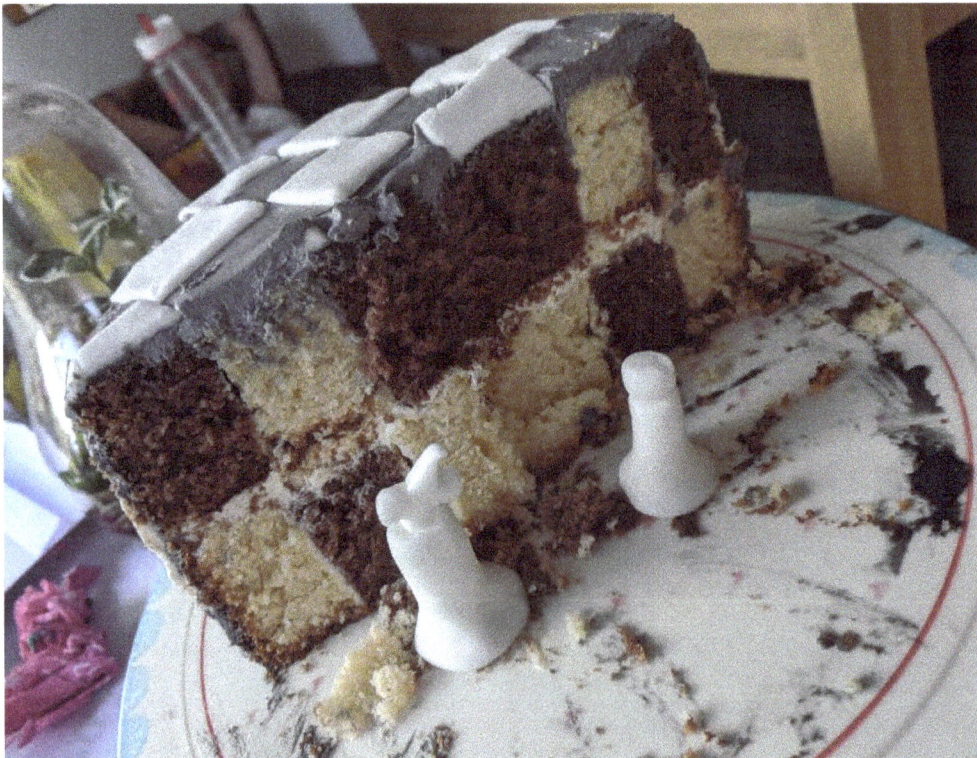

MUG CAKE

(Microwave)

4 tbsp self-raising flour

4 tbsp caster sugar

2 tbsp cocoa powder

1 medium egg

3 tbsp milk

3 tbsp sunflower oil

A few drops vanilla extract

2 tbsp chocolate chips

Method

Use the largest mug. Mix all the ingredients except the choc chip which you put in last. Cook on high for 3/4 mins.

NOTE

Pictures of cakes on the previous page: Pink colouring is pomegranate seeds juiced and for grey in checker cake it is charcoal tablets.

GOLDEN SYRUP CAKE

225g butter

225g sugar

450g golden syrup

450g self-raising flour

2 large eggs

300 ml milk

4 tbsp golden syrup

Method *Bake 50min/140C*

Melt butter, syrup, and sugar for 10 minutes. Beat the eggs with the milk, add the flour and milk/egg mixture to the cooled syrup mixture in the pan and beat until smooth. When baked leave to cool then put extra golden syrup over the top.

BAKED PAPAYA

1 medium peeled, sliced, papaya

1/2 lime juice

vanilla ice cream

Method Bake 180C

Place papaya slices on a non-stick baking sheet. Sprinkle with juice and bake for 15 minutes. Serve: with 1/4 cup ice cream and serve.

PAPAYA MOUSSE

1 papaya, peeled and de-seeded

225 ml double cream

1 vanilla pod, seeds only

2 tbsp caster sugar

55g butter

Method

Mousse

Blend papaya to a purée. Whip the cream together with the vanilla until stiff peaks form. Fold in the puréed papaya and chill.

Butterscotch sauce: Heat the caster sugar in a frying pan and stir in the butter when melted, stir in the cream.

Cook until the sauce thickens and turns a golden-brown colour. Serve: spoon butterscotch sauce into the base of a glass and fill up with the papaya mousse.

ALL IN ONE CAKE

225g butter

225g caster sugar

4 large eggs

225g self-raising flour

2 level tsp baking powder

1 tsp vanilla extract

Method *Bake 180C /25min/*

Combine the dry then wet ingredients into a large bowl and mix well. Place mixture in 20 cm greased tins.

Alternatively, I use this as a basis for other cakes, for example: I just take out the vanilla and put in maple syrup or lime.

Taste great every time.

RED VELVET CAKE

300ml sunflower oil

500g plain flour

2 tbsp cocoa powder

4 tsp baking powder

2 tsp bicarbonate of soda

560g light brown soft sugar

1 tsp fine salt

400ml buttermilk

4 tsp vanilla extract

30ml red food coloring gel Dr Oetker

4 large eggs

For the icing

250g pack unsalted butter 750g icing sugar

350g tub full-fat soft cheese

1 tsp vanilla extract

Method Bake 180C/30mins

Do four sponge cakes in total. Grease two 20cm cake tins.

Mix flour, cocoa, baking powder, bicarbonate of soda, brown sugar, and salt. Then, mix eggs, buttermilk, oil, vanilla extract, 100ml water and 15ml food coloring in a jug.

Pour the wet ingredients into the dry and mix well. Evenly, put the cake mixture into the two tins, and bake.

Icing: Blend butter and half icing sugar until smooth then add the cheese and vanilla and remaining icing sugar and mix.

Icing the Cake

Spread a generous amount of icing on each layer of cake. Keep enough to cover the top and sides of the cake and blend with a knife dipped in warm water.

Can be left in the fridge for two days. Alternative: place cookie in the middle layer.

Tips: My son Peter who made this cake used Dr Oetker red, pink, green. I could not eat the green, so I just took it off my slice.

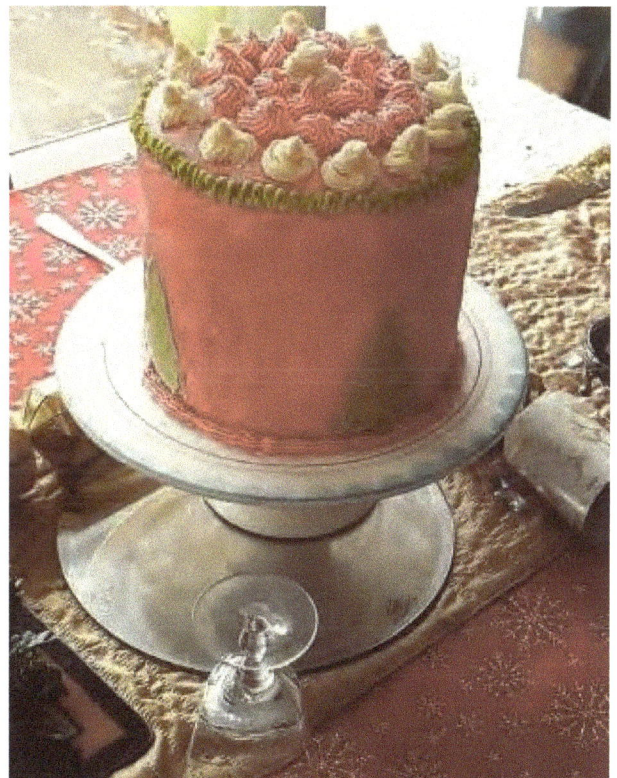

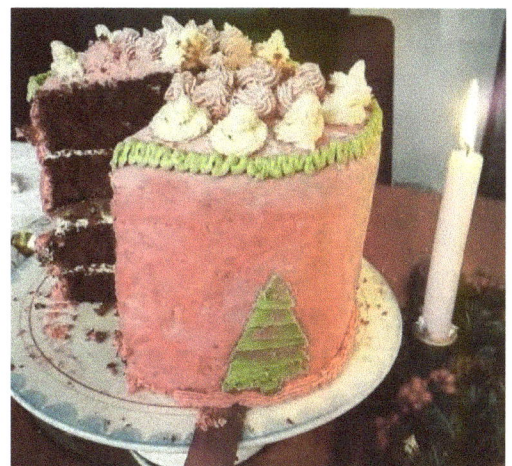

SIMPLE BANANA CAKE

125g butter

150g caster sugar

1 tsp vanilla extract

1 egg, beaten

2 very ripe bananas, mashed

190g self-raising flour

60 ml milk

Method *Bake in Oven 170 C / 35 minutes / Serves: 10 / loaf tin*

Melt the butter, sugar, and vanilla, remove from heat, and add mashed banana. Allow to cool then add the egg, flour, milk and mix well. Pour tin and sprinkle with sugar and bake.

BUTTERSCOTCH PUDDING

200g self-raising flour

175g brown sugar

1 tsp baking powder

100g butter, melted

1 beaten egg

125 ml milk

60g golden syrup

375 ml boiling water

Double cream or ice cream, to serve

Method *Bake 180C / 45 minutes*

Mix 65g of brown sugar flour and baking powder in a bowl and add melted butter, egg, milk and 30g of golden syrup and pour into a greased baking tray.

Syrup: mix 110g of brown sugar and sprinkle over the pudding mixture. Combine boiling water with the remaining 30g of golden syrup. Pour over the top of the pudding mixture and bake.

COFFEE CAKE

225g caster sugar

225g soft unsalted butter

200g plain flour

4 tsp decaf coffee

2 tsp baking powder

4 large eggs

2 tbsp milk

50g pecans nuts

Method Bake 180C/25min

Blitz sugar and pecan add to dry ingredients. Then add butter, eggs, into a large bowl and mix well. Use the milk if necessary. Place mixture in 20 cm greased tins and bake.

POPPY CAKE

50g poppy seeds

185ml warm milk

220g caster sugar

3 eggs

300g self-raising flour

1 tsp baking powder

pinch of salt

200g butter

I tsp vanilla extract

300g icing sugar

Method Bake *180°C/15 minutes*

Combine the poppy seeds and milk in a bowl and set aside for 15 minutes. Mix caster sugar, butter, eggs, and vanilla. Fold in the flour gradually, alternate with the poppy seed and milk mix. Bake in oven till golden brown. Alternative: use all in one cake and add poppy seeds Serve with icing sugar on top.

PEAR CRUMBLE

250g plain flour

90g caster sugar

1 pinch salt

125g salted butter

For the filling

125g sugar

100 ml of water

1 lime, juiced

10 pears or 2 can pears in syrup (omit water)

Method Bake 30mins/ 200 C

Briefly boil the water, sugar, pears chunk together then add the lime juice. Spoon into dish. Mix flour, caster sugar, and butter until the mixture resembles fine breadcrumbs. Cover pears with the crumble topping. Bake until brown.

Alternatively: topping:

1 tbsp of flour

625g rolled oats

200ml pure maple syrup

1 teaspoon baking soda

1 tablespoon rice bran oil

Topping, mix flour, oats, sugar, baking soda then add the oil and mix until crumbly, spread over pears mixture. Drizzle with syrup and bake, serve with cashews on top.

PECAN PIE

15g plain flour

150g butter, melted

150g light brown soft sugar

4 tbsp caster sugar

2 eggs

15g milk

1 tsp vanilla extract

125g chopped pecans

Pastry case (see pastry recipe)

Method *Bake 40min 200C*

Combine eggs and stir in melted butter add sugar's, flour, mix well. Lastly add the milk, vanilla, and pecans. Line tin with pastry and pour filling into base and bake.

APPLE PECAN CAKE

3 cups plain flour

1 tsp baking soda

1 tsp salt

1 cup unsalted butter, melted

2 cups dark brown sugar (packed)

3 large eggs

2 tsp vanilla extract

450 golden delicious apples

225g pecan halves

Method 200C Bake1hr

Sift flour, baking soda, and salt together. Beat butter, sugar, eggs, and vanilla in large mixer bowl until creamy. Stir in dry ingredients. (Batter will be very thick.) Fold in apples, pecans. and pour into prepared tin and cook.

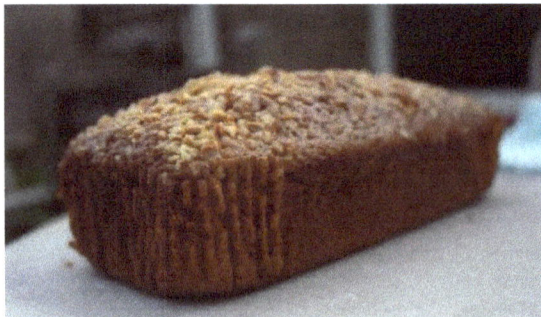

RICE CRISPY BAKE

60g butter

3 tbsp golden syrup

100g bar milk chocolate

90g rice krispies

Method Melt the chocolate in a bowl over a saucepan of simmering water. Mix in the butter and syrup. Remove from heat and add the rice krispies. Spoon into 12 bun cases. Leave to cool.

LIME CHEESECAKE

250g all-butter biscuits (shortbread)

50g butter, melted

40g Icing sugar

250g Philadelphia original or mascarpone cheese

125 ml fresh lime juice

Method

Mix crushed biscuits and butter. Place in 8 ins tin. Mix mascarpone, icing lime juice. Spread over base and chill for 30 minutes. Serve.

CHOCOLATE WEETABIX FUDGE

250g flour

2 tbsp cocoa

4 Weetabix, crushed

2 tsp baking powder

125g sugar

225g butter or spread, melted

60 ml milk

Method *Bake 180C 25 minutes*

Mix dry ingredients, add melted buttermilk. Bake in tray. Ice with chocolate icing. Set in fridge.

APPLE PECAN CRUMBLE

1.5k g golden delicious apples

250 ml water

25g brown sugar

crumble:

125 gr self-raising flour

75g butter

pinch of salt

110g brown sugar

100 porridge oats

50g pecans crushed

4 tbsp maple syrup

Method *Bake 60 minutes / 180C*

Apples: Place peeled, cored, and sliced apples into a pan with sugar, water cook for 10 minutes. Transfer to a shallow ovenproof pie dish.

Crumbles: Blend the flour and butter until the mixture looks like breadcrumbs. Then, add sugar, oats, salt, and nuts. Sprinkle mixture over apples and drizzle with syrup. Bake until golden brown and bubbling.

Serve: with thick cream or custard.

APPLE PIE

12 medium golden delicious apples

125g caster sugar

1 egg

Pastry base (see basic)

Method Bake for 40-45 mins/190C

Slice the apple mix with sugar and lay evenly on the baking sheet. (or stew for minutes with sugar).

After the pastry has chilled, grease a 28cm tin and blind bake pastry for 15 minutes.

Then place in apples and lay the pastry lid over the apples. Brush it all with the egg white and sprinkle with caster sugar bake until golden.

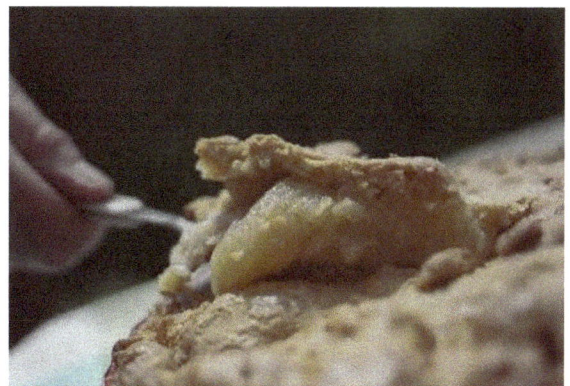

PEAR UPSIDE DOWN CAKE

4 Pears

125g Butter

2 Eggs

450g Self Raising Flour

280g Light Soft Brown Sugar

250ml yoghurt

juice of lime

vanilla extract

Method 180C-45 mins

Melt 125g sugar and 50g butter pour into a 20cm square cake tin. Place pears on top. In a bowl sift the flour

In a bowl mix the eggs with the remaining sugar, lime, and vanilla, mix in melted butter along with the yoghurt.

Pour this mix into the flour and mix well. Pour over the fruit and bake. When cooked and cooled placing a plate or cake stand on top of it turn the whole thing upside on plate.

FRENCH APPLE TART

6 golden delicious apples, finely chopped

60g unsalted butter, cut into small pieces

juice of 1 lime

75g granulated sugar, or to taste

6 tbsp Crème Pâtissière

For the topping:

juice of 1 lime

2 golden delicious thinly sliced

40g butter, melted

Method 180°C bake 30 minutes.

Butter a 22cm tin. See pastry section. Line tin with the rolled-out pastry and bake for 15 minutes. Cook apples in one tablespoon of water for about 20 minutes. Add the butter and sugar lime then set aside to cool. Spread the crème pâtissière in the bottom of the pastry case forming a thin layer followed by apple puree.

Topping: glace the lime juice and apple slices in a shallow bowl and cover with water to prevent the apple discolouring. Drain off lime juice arrange apples on top of the purée in a spiral pattern.

Brush the top of the apple slices with the melted butter and bake the tart in an oven preheated to

Glaze: use some of the apple syrup when the tart's done, lightly brush, over the hot tart in the direction of the apple slices and set aside to cool.

TWO WAY CHESSY SCONES

350g self-raising flour

100g English cheddar grated

150 ml fresh milk

75g butter

1 egg beaten

Method *Use for Cobbler topping for a casserole or a batch of delicious scones*

Rub the butter into the flour until like fine breadcrumbs and then stir in cheese. Add egg and milk and mix to a dough.

Ploughman Lunch

Bake 230C / 10-15minutes

Roll scones as above. Place on a tray in the oven, bake. Serve hot with a side salad.

Cobbler topping: Roll dough to 1cm of 8 rounds. Twenty minutes before the end of the casserole set oven to 230 C. Remove lid place scones on top and continue baking until scones have risen.

SCONES

450g self-raising flour, plus more for dusting

half tsp salts

1 tsp baking powder

120g butter cut into cubes

60g caster sugar

milk as required

1 tsp vanilla extract

squeeze lime juice

3 eggs beaten -to glaze

clotted cream, to serve

Method Bake 15 mins

Mix flour the salt and baking powder, add the butter, then mix until it looks like fine crumbs.

Stir in the sugar and add milk, vanilla, and lime juice. Combine liquid with flour mixture with a knife. On flour work surface knead the dough and make into use a 5cm cutter. Brush the tops with beaten egg place on baking tray cook until golden brown.

CHOCOLATE BROWNIE

250g plain flour

400g milk chocolate, chopped

280g butter

350g brown sugar

6 eggs

Method *Bake /180°C/35 minutes/Serves 8.*

Place half the chocolate and butter in a small saucepan over low heat and stir until melted and smooth then allow to cool slightly.

Combine sugar, eggs, and flour in a bowl with the chocolate mixture and stir through the remaining chocolate pieces then pour the mixture into a lightly greased 20cm x 30cm tin lined with non-stick baking paper and bake.

Alternatives using this mixture make: brownie cupcakes - divide the mixture between 12 x muffin tins lined with paper cases and bake for 30 minutes. Spread brownie cashew butter frosting over cupcakes to serve.

SCOTCH

100g caster sugar

200g flour (plain or self-raising)

2 egg

20 ml milk or as required

Method Makes /12 pancakes

Mix the flour and sugar, egg together and add milk as required. Make a thick, smooth batter.

When the frying pan is hot, ladle in some of the batters. Pancake is ready to be turned when it bubbles. Turn and cook until the surface is golden brown.

SHORTBREAD BISCUITS

250g butter

110g caster sugar, plus extra to finish

360g plain flour

Method *Bake 15mins180C*

*Make 24*Combine all the ingredients in a bowl. Roll the mixture into a ball, flatten and place on baking tray and bake.

OAT BISCUITS

75g plain flour

1 tsp baking powder

75g porridge oats

75g sugar

75g butter

20 ml golden syrup

20 ml milk

Method Bake 180C/15mins

Mix flour, baking powder, porridge oats, and sugar together. Melt butter, syrup, and milk in a saucepan and add to the premixed dry ingredients. Shape into rounds and place them on the baking tray. Bake until golden brown. Leave to cool for 5 minutes before removing

FOUR TYPES OF BISCUITS

100g butter

100g caster sugar

225g self-raising flour sugar

1 egg

Method Bake for 20 ins at 190c./ (24 biscuits)

Cream butter, sugar until fluffy and gradually add egg and fold in the flour. Divide mixture into four. Fold one of the flavours into the dough and then roll into walnut size balls and put on the tray.

Chocolate: Dissolve 2 tbsp cocoa in 1 tsp hot water and fold into mixture.

Cashew (or pecan or hazelnut)

Fold 2 tsp of crushed nuts into mixture.

Citrus: Juice of 1 lime and fold in. Poppy seeds: Fold 2 tsp poppy seeds in the mixture.

GOLDEN SYRUP FLAPJACKS

250g rolled oats (porridge oats)

125g butter

125g Brown sugar

50g Golden Syrup

Method *Bake 180C,25 minutes*

Makes 12-16 Put the butter, sugar and golden syrup and gently heat until melted. Stir in the oats and mix. Turn into the tin and bake.

VANILLA WAFERS

250g self-raising flour

1 tsp baking powder

125g unsalted butter, room temperature

125g ounces vanilla sugar

20 ml vanilla extract

20 ml whole milk

1 large egg

salt

Method *Bake 200C/ 20 minutes*

Sift together the flour, baking powder, and salt in a small bowl and set aside. Cream the butter and vanilla sugar in the bowl for 2 minutes. Add the egg, vanilla extract and milk and blend on low speed for 15 seconds and add the flour mixture.

Chill the batter in the refrigerator for at least 10 minutes. Scoop the batter in teaspoon-sized balls and arrange them on 2 parchments paper-lined approximately 35 cookies per pan and flatten each ball the bake.

BAKED PAPAYA

1 medium peeled, sliced, papaya

1/2 lime juice

vanilla ice cream

Method Bake 180C

Place papaya slices on a non-stick baking sheet. Sprinkle with juice and bake for 15 minutes.

Serve: top each slice with 1/4 cup ice cream and serve.

CHOCOLATE BUTTERCREAM ICING

Chocolate buttercream icing

100g milk chocolate

200g butter softened

400g icing sugar

5 tbsp cocoa powder

2 tbsp milk

Method

Put the chocolate in a heatproof bowl over a pan of barely simmering water. Stir until melted then mix the butter and icing sugar together.

Sift in the cocoa and pour in the melted chocolate, a pinch of salt and the milk, then mix again until smooth. Use to top cupcakes or cover and fill a chocolate sponge cake.

VANILLA MASCARPONE CAKE *FILLER*

450g mascarpone cheese, at room temperature

250ml heavy cream

100g granulated sugar

Seeds scraped from 1 vanilla bean, or 2 tsp. pure vanilla extract

Pinch table salt

Method

Mix cream, sugar, vanilla seeds or extract, and salt and beat until the mixture is thick and holds firm peaks, but don't overbeat or the frosting will look grainy.

CARMEL SYRUP SAUCES

250g brown sugar

125g butter

80 ml milk

pinch salt

1 tsp vanilla extract

Method

Bring brown sugar, butter, and milk to a gentle boil and cook until thickened, 2 minutes.

Remove from heat, add vanilla extract, cool slightly and pour the sauce into a jar.

Serve: refrigerate until cold.

MAPLE CARAMEL SAUCE

125g unsalted butter

500g brown sugar

250g pure maple syrup

1/2 tsp. salt

Method

Makes about 3 cups

Melt butter add sugar and salt and cook until sugar is completely dissolved, then boil for 2 minutes. Add maple syrup and boil for 2 to 4 minutes.

Serve: cool pour into containers and refrigerate will keep for up to 2 months.

BUTTERSCOTCH SAUCE

160 ml single cream

155g brown sugar

50g butter, cubed

2 tsp vanilla essence

Method

Place the cream, sugar, butter, and vanilla extract in a pot and stir until well mixed. Then increase heat to high and bring to the boil. Reduce heat to simmer, uncovered for 5 minutes or until the sauce thickens slightly.

Serve: leave to cool then serve.

FUDGE ICING

170g condensed milk

100g butter mis

100g chocolate

Method

Melt over simmering water. Cool the spread over cake.

BUTTER CREAM FROSTING

350g of icing sugar

175g soft unsalted butter

2 tsp instant decaf coffee (dissolved in 1 tbsp boiling water)

approx. 10 pecans (to decorate)

Method

Sieve the icing sugar and beat it into the butter with a wooden spoon. Then beat in the hot coffee liquid. Spread in middle and top with a swirly pattern on top and nuts around sides. Good with coffee cake

CASHEW BUTTER FROSTING

140g smooth cashew butter

50g unsalted butter softened

250 ml pouring cream, whipped to soft peaks

80g icing sugar

1 tsp vanilla extract

60 ml single cream

Method

Combine cashew or hazelnut butter, sugar, butter, and vanilla and beat until light and fluffy. Add the cream and beat for 2 minutes. Spread over the cake to serve.

SWEET RICOTTA TOPPING

200g ricotta cheeses or cottage chess -sieved

400 ml whipping cream

30 ml of maple syrup (or golden syrup)

15 ml lime juice

1 tsp. vanilla

Method

Place ricotta, syrup, lime juice and vanilla in food processor container cover. Process until smooth. Place in a bowl and add whipped topping stir until well blended. Cover.

Serve: refrigerate at least 1 hour before serving. Great for cheesecake and pancake filling.

CRÈME PATISSIERE

Pastry Cream

4 egg yolks

100g caster sugar

30g plain flour

3 tbsp corn starch

350 ml whole milk

2 vanilla beans, split and seeded, or 1 teaspoon pure vanilla extract

Method

Whisk together egg yolks and sugar just until pale and creamy, then add and flour.

Heat milk add vanilla bring to the boil. Remove from heat and remove vanilla bean. Gradually pour the hot milk into the egg mixture, whisk until smooth.

Transfer mixture back into saucepan. Cook, whisking constantly, so that the eggs won't curdle, simmer for 1 minute until mixture thickens.

Sieve and allow to cool. Cover with cling film touching to prevent it from creating a skin. Cool, refrigerate, can use up to 3 days.

BASIC RECIPES

SIMPLE BATTER

250g self-raising flour

2 tsp butter, melted (optional)

250g soda water or plain water

1 pinch salt

Method

Whisk the melted butter flour, salt, and then add soda water. The lumps will disappear while frying.

Flour and water batter: Beat 250gr flour and of salt into 250mls of water. Set aside to rest for 30 minutes before using.

Baking Powder Batter: When you want a crunchy crust. Stir flour, 2 teaspoons of baking powder and salt together whisk in 250mls of water until smooth. Serve: use immediately.

EGG WHITE BATTER

250g flour

1tsp salt

250 ml water

3 eggs

cream of tartar

Method: Mix flour, salt with 250mls of cold water until smooth. Set aside and let rest for at least 30 minutes. Beat 3 egg whites with a pinch of cream of tartar until they form medium peaks. Gently fold the whites into the flour-water mix. Serve: use immediately.

Tips -To make a crispy batter you need to get air in mixture. There are two methods for doing so: adding a raising agent, such as baking powder or yeast or making up the batter with a soda water /carbonated liquid.

YORKSHIRE PUDDING

85g plain flour

85g milk

65g water

1 egg

Method Bake/200 c/20 minutes

Put on tray equal parts of butter and sunflower oil just enough to cover the bottom. Put into the oven.

GARLIC BUTTER

125g butter

2 garlic cloves, minced

2 tbsp fresh chopped chives

Salt to taste

Method

Mix all ingredients into a bowl Garlic butter will last about a week in the fridge or in put in the freezer in an ice cube tray.

PASTRY

225g plain flour

135g butter

2 tsps. icing sugar(optional)

1 egg yolk, beaten with 1 tsp cold water

Method

Mix all the pastry ingredients together to form a soft dough. Set aside to rest for 30 minutes in fridge. Roll as desired.

EASY WHITE SAUCE

250 ml cream

250 ml milk

50g butter

50g flour

Method

Boil milk, cream, and butter together. Then add flour and beat continuously until creamy and thick. Cook garlic in butter for 1 minute and add to the sauce and simmer for 5 minutes.

Chesses sauce

Take off the heat, then stir in 250g grated mature cheddar and 25g grated parmesan.

CARAMELISED ONION SAUCE

1 tbsp sunflower oil or butter

8 medium-sized shallots, *very thinly sliced (about 5 cups)*

1/2 teaspoon salt

Method

Fry shallots in oil for two minutes, add salt, stirring occasionally, for 10 minutes.

Put on low heat, cover, and cook from 30 to 45 minutes longer.

This sauce is very versatile and is used on pasta or homemade pizza etc.

It can be stored in a fridge for one week.

GREEK YOGURT WITH PECANS

25g pecans, roughly chopped

300g Greek yogurt

4 tsp maple syrup

Method *Serves 2*

Lightly toast the pecans and set aside to cool. Put the yoghurt into two bowls, throw in nuts on top, drizzle with maple syrup.

Serve immediately.

RICE CRISPY STUFFING

750g rice krispies

750g breadcrumbs or bran flakes

125 shallots chopped

125 diced celery

1 tsp salt

1 egg, well beaten

125g butter, melted

125g milk

Method *Bake/180c/20 minutes*

Combine rice krispies, breadcrumbs, shallots, celery and salt, egg, butter, and milk. Mix well.

BRAN FLAKE STUFFING

125ml maple syrup

bran flakes

1 clove garlic

30g butter

1 tsp lime

Method *Bake/180c/20 minutes*

Combine in a pot, heat until bubbling then transfer to oven.

GREEK HUMMUS

DIPS

440g chickpeas (garbanzos), drained and rinsed

2 cloves garlic, crushed

3 tbsp sunflower oil

1/3 tsp citric acid

salt to taste

Method

Combine ingredients in the food processor and blend until smooth.

ALTERNATIVE HUMMUS

440g chickpeas, drained

2 cloves garlic

40g poppy seeds

half tsp salts

Juice of 1 lime

6 tbsp sunflower oil

Method

Toast the poppy seeds and hazelnuts in a pan on low heat until they brown lightly. In a food processor blend into fine powder add chickpeas and the remaining hummus ingredients until smooth.

Serve Garnish-small handful of hazelnuts nuts and a drizzle of oil. transfer to a plate to serve.

CASHEW SAUCE

2 cups cashews

350 ml water or broth

2 cloves garlic

1 tsp salt

Method

Soak cashews in a bowl for 2 hours. Drain and rinse thoroughly then put in a food processor with water, garlic, and salt.

Puree until very, very smooth. Thin out with more water to desired consistency.

Serve: store in the fridge for 4 days or freeze.

For pasta, dips, or cheesy sauce alternatives.

PEA SAUCE

500g frozen peas

20g butter

1 medium shallot chopped

2 garlic cloves, crushed

60g pure cream

Method

Cook peas in a saucepan of boiling water for 2 to 3 minutes or until tender. Drain.

Melt butter adds shallot and garlic and cook, stirring for 3 minutes or until softened. Return peas to pan add cream. Cook for 1 minute or until heated through, blend. Serve- goes well with Lamb fillet

QUICK PEAR CHUTNEY

3 large pears, chopped small

2 medium shallots finely chopped

160 ml rice vinegar

60g soft brown sugar

pinch of sea salt

Method

Add the ingredients to the pot and simmer, stirring to dissolve the sugar. Simmer without the lid for about 20 minutes until most of the liquid has evaporated. Spoon the chutney into a hot sterilised jar and seal. It can be stored in the fridge or frozen.

SATAY SAUCE

1 tbsp golden syrup or maple syrup

2 tbsp cashew nut butter

20g butter

1 clove garlic, crushed

salt to taste

Method

Melt butter in a saucepan over low heat, and stir in other ingredients until mixed, pour remaining sauce over rice. Serve: This mock-peanut sauce goes well with chicken satay and rice.

MASCARPONE CHEESE SAUCE

250g mascarpone cheese

125g butter

125g grated Parmesan cheese (or cheddar)

25g hazelnuts or pecan nuts

heavy cream (as needed)

Method

Melt butter then adds mascarpone cheese until melted follow with parmesan cheese. Finely add nuts and if needed, adjust the sauce's thickness with heavy cream.

SHALLOT DRESSING

2 shallots

15 ml rice vinegar

10 ml soft brown sugar

30 ml sunflower oil

Salt

Method

Combine the shallots, vinegar, sugar, salt and leave for about an hour. Then add the oil and stir well. Use this with lentils, topped with goat's cheese or feta.

QUICK SALAD DRESSING

A bunch of chives

1 garlic clove, crushed

100 ml sunflower oil

A pinch of salt

Method

Blend all ingredients together

HOISIN DIPPING SAUCE

60g soy sauce

30g smooth cashew butter

15g brown sugar

2 tsp rice wine vinegar

1 garlic clove, finely minced

2 tsp sunflower oil

125g dark Miso paste, such as brown rice

Method

Put all the ingredients into a blender and blitz to a smooth liquid.

PEAR SAUCE

4 ripe pears peeled, chopped

1 celery

150 ml water

1 tbsp of lime juice

25g butter

2 tbsp caster sugar

Method

Heat the butter and sizzle the pear chunks, celery together until brown. Add water, lime, and sugar. Cook until it becomes sticky and caramelised mash pears if necessary.

SALAD CREAM

20g sugar

50 ml malt vinegar

50 ml of cream

salt

Method Mix well store in the fridge.

LIME BUTTER SAUCE

2 garlic chopped

85 ml fresh lime juice

1 tsp salt

125g butter, melted

Method

Purée garlic with lime juice, salt, and butter. Serve: can be refrigerated.

SOY LIME SAUCE

1 clove garlic

50g sugar

85g soy sauce

50g fresh lime juice

65 ml water, or to taste

Method

Blend garlic, sugar, soy sauce, lime juice, and water. Stir until well blended.

Serve: this sauce will keep up to 3 weeks if stored in the refrigerator.

LIME DRESSING

15 ml lime juice

45 ml sunflower oil

Salt

Method

Whisk together, taste and adjust seasoning.

PEAR JAM

1 kg ripe pears cut into small pieces

60 ml of filtered water

1 tsp of vanilla extract

200 ml of rice malt syrup or maple syrup

50g packet of Jamsetta

Alternative

Replace fresh pears with 2 tin of pears.

Chokoes can be used instead of pears.

Method

Place chopped pears into the pot with water, vanilla and syrup. Cook 20 minutes or until very soft.

Puree and then mix in Jamsetta and cook for about ten minutes. Allow to cool and pour into sterile jars.

Refrigerate or freeze. Use within 10 days of opening

Boiling fruit causes them to increase in salicylates so only the peers and chokoes can be used.

JAPANESE STYLE SAUCE

6 sticks of celery chopped

3 large apples,

small head red cabbage,

30g Miso

750 ml of water.

4 cloves garlic

chives

2 tbsp arrowroot, dissolve in 85mls water

Miso (fermented bean paste) is a concentrated, savoury paste.

Method

Bake 40 mins/Serves 8 people

Place all ingredients in boiling water, boil until very soft. Arrowroot can be added for extra sheen and body.

Simmer for 20 minutes, allowing the flavour to improve. Adjust seasoning to taste.

BLACK BEAN SAUCE

30g sunflower oil

180g salted black beans, drained & rinsed

4 cloves garlic, chopped

200 ml water

2 tbsp dark soy sauce

4 tbsp rice wine

2 tsp sugar

2-3 tsp cornflour

Method

Heat the oil and add the beans and garlic and cook for a few minutes. Mix the remaining ingredients then add to the pan. Bring up to the boil, stirring. When thickened, the sauce is read.

Serve: use or allow to cool, bottle, and refrigerate for later.

Use for – Chicken Chow Mein

SILKEN TOFU DRESSING

60g soft tofu

1 tsp sunflower or bran oil

60 ml lime juice

10 ml maple syrup

50g raw cashew nuts chopped

1 tbs sweet miso

Method

Place tofu in blender or food processor and blend until smooth. Then add remaining ingredients and blend.

Keeps in fridge for 1 week

Silken tofu becomes a creamy base for almost any kind of sauce, dressing, or dip.

MAYONNAISE

1 tin condensed milk (395 Grams)

250 ml malt vinegar

Salt

Method

Pour condensed milk into a bowl with salt and slowly whisk in the malt vinegar. Use right away or refrigerate until needed.

FAKE TOMATO SAUCE

TOMATOES substitute for pizza, see under sauces:

caramelized onion sauce

fake tomato sauce

cashew sauce

Break down the components of tomatoes and consider alternatives.

Water: tomatoes are just wet, so you'll need some liquid.

Sugar: tomatoes are naturally sweet, so you'll need some sugar/maple syrup Acid: malt vinegar or lime juice, citric acid Seasoning's: shallots, garlic, salt, chives.

FAKE TOMATO SAUCE RECIPE

250g red kidney beans, rinsed

2 large pear halves in syrup

250 ml of water

1 tsp citric acid

165g white sugar

1 tsp salt

1 stick Celery (trimmed and chopped)

4 Spring onions (chopped)

3 tsp crushed garlic

10 Saffron threads (soaked in a bit of water)

Method

Place all the ingredients into a saucepan on low heat. Cover and simmer for 30 minutes until. Remove from the heat and allow to cool slightly.

Then pour into a food processor and blend until very smooth. Return the sauce to the saucepan. If the sauce is a bit thick add some more water. Allow simmering for 15 minutes. Storage put into sterilised jars and seal, store in the fridge in an airtight container for about 2 weeks.

Recipe from: www.cookingforoscar.com/recipe/no-tomato-sauce

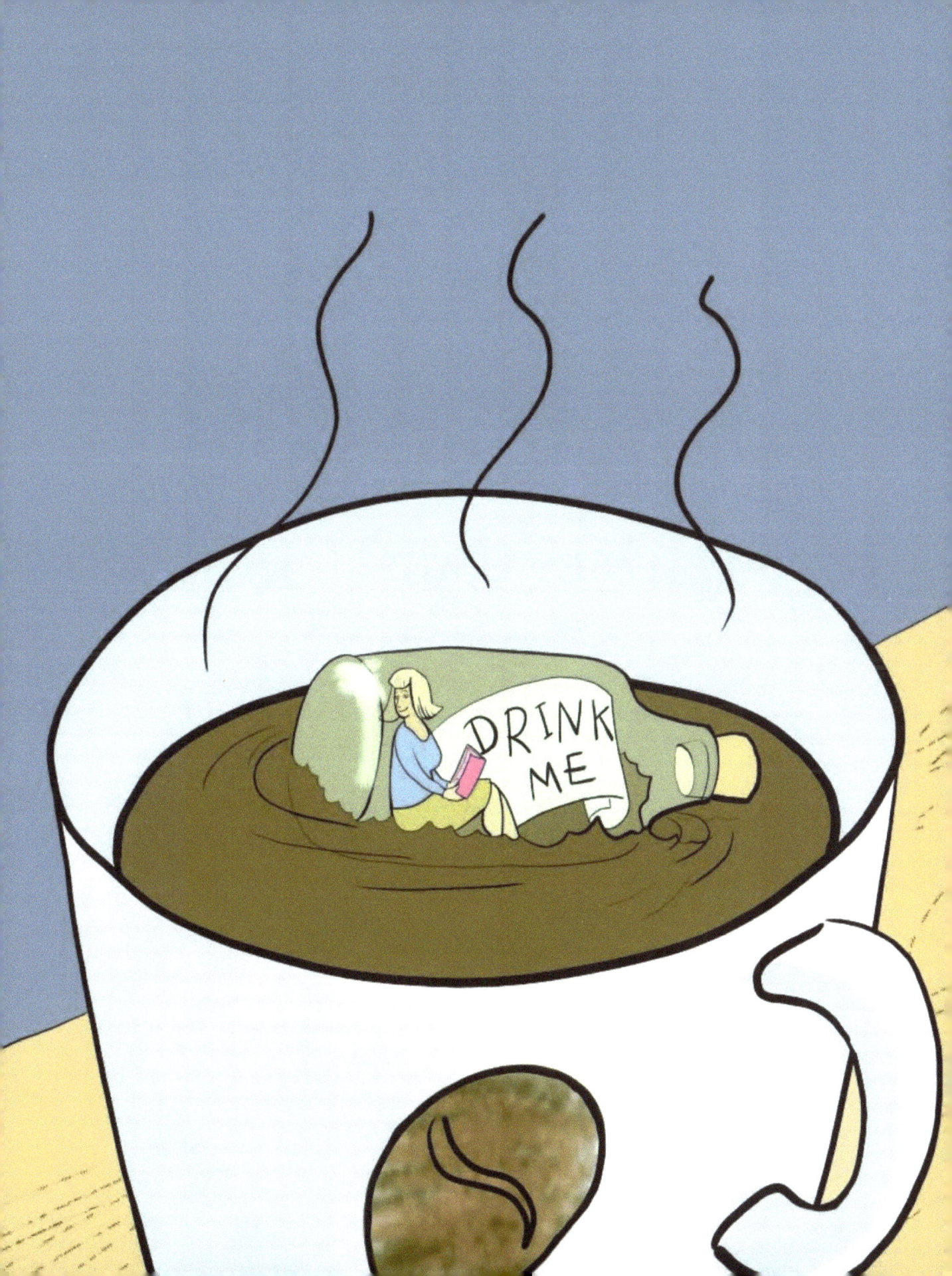

BEVERAGES

SIMPLE PEAR JUICE

8 large ripe pears

1500 ml of water

125g sugar

Method

Peel pears cut into cubes. Place into a deep cooking pot. Add lime to the pot. Add sugar and water and stir everything.

Bring to boil, simmer for 10-15 minutes, or until pears are very soft.

Cooldown to room temperature. Blend until smooth. Store in the fridge for up to 5 days.

PEAR NECTAR

6 fully ripped pears, chopped

30 ml lime juice

1250 ml of water

tbsp maple syrup

Method Cook 20 minutes/Yield: 1 litre

Place pears into the saucepan and cover with water, simmer for 15 minutes.

Puree, then fine sieve. Serve: put into jar or bottle in the refrigerator until ready to use.

It can also be used on desserts.

BANANA CREAM PIE SMOOTHIE

2 bananas, sliced and frozen

250 ml milk

1/3 cup low-fat vanilla Greek yoghurt

2 tsp vanilla extract

4 vanilla wafer cookies (See page)

25g maple syrup

250g rice

Method

Place all ingredients in the body of a blender. Pulse until smooth and creamy and serve.

OLD FASHION LEMONADE

500 ml of water

500g sugar,1 tsp citric acid

Method

Place water and sugar in a 1-pint jug and heat in the microwave for 2 minutes. Stir the sugar until

dissolved and then add citric acid. Dilute to taste with water or soda water.

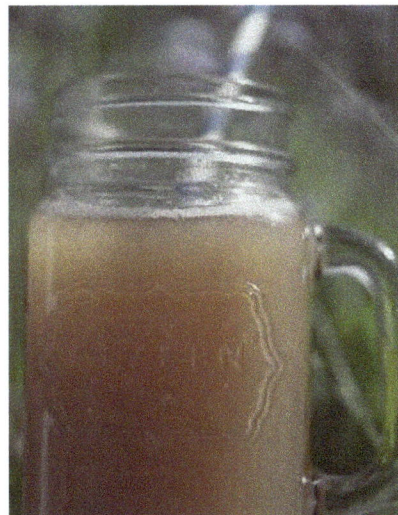

CELERY SMOOTHIE

3 stalks of organic celery

250 ml of water

Method

Put into a blender, add water, pulse until smooth, serve.

QUICK APPLE JUICE

4 golden delicious

250 ml water

Optional- half small lime

Method

Peel core and slice apples. Add to blender with other ingredients and then strain and serve.

APPLE JUICE PUREE

18 Apples

Optional- sugar

Method

Core, peel apples cut into slices, add water to cover them. Boil apples for 25 minutes. Sieve add additional sugar if necessary or add water if too strong.

Leftover apple mush can be turned into apple sauce by puréeing.

Keep it refrigerated use it within a week.

LIME DRINK

250 ml fresh lime juice, chilled

30g caster sugar

1-litre soda water, chilled

Ice cubes, to serve

half tsp salts

Lime wedges, to serve

Method

Combine the lime juice, salt, and sugar in a large jug and stir well until the sugar and salt dissolve. Add soda water and stir to combine.

Place the ice cubes and lime wedges in glasses and add the lime juice and soda. Serve: immediately.

PAPAYA SMOOTHIES

1 small papaya, peeled, seeded, and diced

1 banana, sliced

lime juice

Method

Combine the papaya, banana and about 15 ice cubes in a blender and purée until smooth.

SIMPLE DAIRY TOFFEE

SWEETS

275g dark brown soft sugar

325g caster sugar

225g butter

350g golden syrup

300 ml double cream

175 ml full-fat milk

2 tsp vanilla extract

Method Serves: 12

Combine dark brown sugar, caster sugar, butter, golden syrup, cream, milk and vanilla in a medium saucepan over medium heat.

Heat, stirring occasionally until a small amount of syrup dropped into cold water forms a rigid ball.

Pour into a 20x20cm tin. Let cool before cutting into small squares.

HOME MADE TOFFEE

250g hazelnuts

250g cup unsalted butter, cubed

250g sugar

1/2 teaspoon vanilla extract

half tsp salts

400g chocolate chips

80g pecans, chopped

Method Bake 190C.

Spread hazelnuts in an even layer onto the prepared baking sheet.

Place into oven and bake for about 10 minutes, set aside. Combine butter, sugar vanilla and salt in a pan over medium heat.

Cook, whisking constantly until butter has melted for about 15 minutes.

Immediately spread the hot caramel mixture evenly over the hazelnuts.

Sprinkle with chocolate chips in an even layer until smooth.

Sprinkle with pecans. Let cool completely, about 2 hours. Break into pieces.

REFERENCES

Just a few of the areas of research for this book

http://www.slhd.nsw.gov.au/rpa/allergy/resources/foodintol/salicylates.html

https://www.histamineintolerance.org.uk/about/the-food-diary/the-food-list/

ttp://www.bmj.com/content/319/7202/90.1

http://foodintolerances.org/intolerances/histamine-biogenic-amines-intolerance/

http://www.feingold.org/Research/pst.php#Corder

https://geneticliteracyproject.org/2017/05/24/lose-energy-eating-brussels-sprouts-taking-aspirin-mystery-behind-salicylate-intolerance/

https://salicylatesensitivity.com/forum/ Salicylates Forum-Support group

https://www.ncbi.nlm.nih.gov/pmc/articles/PMC2995314/ Control of Biogenic Amines in Food

http://allergy.net.au/wp-content/uploads/2013/01/Handbook-p1-33.pdf#page=19&zoom=auto,869,323

https://www.greatplainslaboratory.com/gpl-blog-source/2016/6/6/your-bodys-detoxification-pathways.

http://www.enzymestuff.com/epsomsalts.htm

https://www.drlaurendeville.com/articles/liver-detoxifies/

https://www.eonutrition.co.uk/post/sulfate-i-the-basics

https://www.ncbi.nlm.nih.gov/pubmed/18795922

Research on PST, Salicylates & Sulfation

https://pdfs.semanticscholar.org/e855/35d31622889db45c4d428b4a048d87bc980c.pdf

Significance of salicylates Intolerance in disease of the lower gastrointestinal tract
http://www.eaaci.org/attachments/9c%20-%20raithelSalicylINT.pdf

Sensitivity to food additives, vaso-active amines and salicylates: a review of the evidence

https://www.ncbi.nlm.nih.gov/pmc/articles/PMC4604636/ Control of salicylate intolerance with fish oils. Healy E, Newell.

www.ingramcontent.com/pod-product-compliance
Lightning Source LLC
Chambersburg PA
CBHW042351030426

42336CB00026B/3445